Intermittent Fasting

How to Lose Weight With This Popular Eating Plan

Contents

Introduction

Intermittent fasting is one of the most popular diets out there now a day and why would not it be? People enjoy freedom and unlike every other diet, intermittent fasting offers freedom on what to eat and when to eat. Most diets even have the need of counting calories, but intermittent fasting in general does not require you to count calories.

Intermittent fasting is basically fasting, eating and then fasting again. There are different types of intermittent fasting methods are available. These methods are designed in such a way that everyone can try them. Starting should always be slow and steady, so when you are picking any method, make sure not to challenge yourself too hard at the very beginning.

This book contains a detailed description on what is intermittent diet, how does it work, tips and tricks, food list, meal plan and most importantly the recipes. The recipes are simple and easy to follow. They are divided between breakfast, lunch, dinner, snacks and desserts.

Before starting any diet, one should check with their doctor, so before you start your intermittent fasting journey, make sure to call up your doctor and get their opinion.

What is "Intermittent fasting"?

Intermittent fasting is in the simplest term, fasting for a few days or a period of time and then resuming normal eating. Intermittent fasting is considered to be a very popular diet nowadays, but it does not have the characteristics of a conventional diet! In any other diet, you do eat a certain way in a certain manner, you have a list of foods to avoid and consume. In intermittent fasting, there is no hard and fast rule of choosing what food to eat and not. Intermittent fasting also does not require you to follow a strict time schedule, when you should refrain from eating!

Intermittent fasting can be done by anyone at any time. It does not come up with a rule that you need to do it for a week or a month or 6 months. You can do it for as long as you possibly can, and then if you like it, if your body comprehends the method of eating and gives you benefit, then you would invariably continue the diet. If anyone wants to quit after one week, there is no harm. It does not come with any side effects. You can leave the diet any time you want. So anyone who is reluctant to try the diet because you are afraid you would not be able to continue, don't be scared!

People around the world use intermittent fasting as a tool to lose weight. Most people take it as a challenge, as research has shown intermittent fasting has a significant weight loss value. Some people do intermittent fasting simply to save up time. There are task masters living around you who do not live to eat, but eat to live! They are happy if they could skip meals and with intermittent fasting, their skipping meals become beneficial for them. Some people often try intermittent fasting to remain healthy and fit. Research has shown that people who fast for at least 2 days per week are very active in everything, have better sleep at night, and remain joyous. Intermittent fasting is also used for religious purposes. In Islam people fast for an entire month and they come out feeling better than ever. In Hinduism, Buddhism, Christianity, and Zionism people do intermittent fasting to show tribute to their GOD and to become pure spiritually and physically.

Different Methods of Intermittent Fasting

While intermittent fasting does not come with any restrictions, there are a few methodical differences between each type. There are 6 different ways you can approach the diet. All of the methods are good and proven to help you reach your goals of losing weights, feeling fresh and active, lessen fatigue problems, combat over-eating, get glowing skin, improving metabolism and combat many diseases.

But you know the term,

"One size fits all"

Intermittent fasting does not go by this rule. Intermittent fasting is flexible and as not all body functions the same way, there are different ways intermittent fasting can favor you. No one would be able to guarantee you that one method would work better than the other for you unless you yourself try all the methods. You need to decide after trying them out, which one works well for you. Your body is something you are most familiar with, so if a method works for someone else, it does not mean it will work for you too. You need to go out and do it yourself in order to find your right fit.

Here are the different methods of intermittent fasting,

24 hours intermittent fasting

The method is as simple as the title suggests. You need to refrain from eating for 24 hours straight. In these 24 hours, you would not eat anything. You can of course drink water to stay hydrated. When you are fasting, staying hydrated is very important. You are doing the diet to improve your health, but if you become dehydrated, intermittent fasting can be hazardous for you. So you need to be extra careful during your early days of fasting. You need to constantly drink lots of liquid to stay hydrated. After successfully fasting for entire 24 hours, you can eat anything for the next 4-5 days or more.

Here when we say anything, we literally do not mean anything as it is after all a diet and if you munch on chocolate bars, milkshakes and chips, then what good will the diet bring? It will only bring diarrhea or gestational problems. So stay aware of these things.

If you are staring new, I would suggest do not start straight with 24 hours fast as you would probably faint or feel very stressed. Intermittent fasting is something you need to train your body to with time. 24 hours is not easy and I am not saying it is impossible as of course people have done it in the past and are still doing it today. But people who are accustomed to fasting generally can survive a 24 hours fast. A newbie would feel very anxious and lethargic in the process. You should do 24 hours fast only after you have tried few of the other intermittent fasting methods and see that your body succumbed to it well.

The 16/8 Method

Martin Berkhan, a fitness expert called, the method Leangain protocol. 16/8 intermittent fasting method is when you refrain yourself from eating for 16 hours straight and then allow yourself to eat for the next 8 hours. This type of fasting is done by Muslims during Ramadan as they start their fast with the sunrise and break it with the sundown. They fast for 30 days straight and come out feeling pure and very active. So anyone who is reluctant and questioning about health conditions should not be afraid. Of course you do not need to do 16/8 intermittent fasting for a month, they are doing it for religious purposes. You can do it as often as you feel like doing it or as long as your body is supporting it well.

If you think about it, you probably have done 16/8 fast in your life before. Think of the time you had a very early dinner at 7 pm and waking up straight in the noon or woke up early but skipped breakfast. That way you have already without knowing refrained from eating for 16 hours! Now if you could survive it unknowingly, you can do it when you make a conscious decision of going on a rules free heavenly diet! Now the question of skipping breakfast comes alone if it is unhealthy to skip , this deserves more explanation and I will do it in our upcoming chapters.

12:12 Hours Fasting

This is another convenient option for beginners at intermittent fasting. Here you get a chance to fast for 12 hours and then have the opportunity to eat for the next 12 hours. This intermittent fasting method is rather easy and does not give you any hunger pans. Most people don't even feel they are doing anything differently. Just skipping breakfast or skipping dinner is enough to try this method of intermittent fasting. It is much easier to fast everyday when you use this method.

5:2 Diet

5:2 fasting method is very popular for losing weight and more people are choosing it as it gives them time to eat as they like for 5 days and they have to stick to a 500-600 calories per day for 2 days a week. You yourself would decide which food you would eat and drink, that just needs to be within 500-600 calories. Food requirements are different in men and women and therefore women have 500 calorie restriction and men have 600 calorie restriction.

The days can be fixed by the dieter. If you are a working person, you can manage the days that are less troubling for you. For one week if you choose Sunday and Tuesday, for the next you can pick Friday or Wednesday, there is no strict guideline on dates either. It can be any 2 days from the week. Give yourself two meals per day, that way you can easily divide the calories. If you want to add in healthy snacks, then make sure you count the calories well.

Dr Michael Mosley termed this diet as the fast diet because of its nature.

Alternate Day Fasting

This method is also challenging for few as it requires to fast for an entire day and then continuing a regular eating pattern the next day. Then continue with fasting for an entire day. This method should be easy for people who are again familiar with intermittent fasting.

The Warrior Diet

The warrior's way of fasting is remaining hungry for the entire day and then eating food at night. This can work well for people who are workaholics and do not have time to eat. This can also be very useful for people who are traveling far. Eating in a journey can be difficult and unwanted for a few people. If you train your body for the warrior diet, then you can easily skip eating during a long journey.

You can however have small portions of fruits and vegetables that are healthy during the day. Do not eat anything heavy though. For the warrior method of fasting, you get a 4 hours window to eat anything during the night.

Since it is called the warrior diet, you also should eat like how our warriors of ancient times used to eat, "unprocessed food". You should only eat foods that are not processed; basically "whole food" is the way to go with this method. Warrior fasting method is quite similar to the food choices we have in the "paleo diet".

Skipping Meal when Convenient

This is the simplest way of doing intermittent fasting. Skip meals whenever possible or whenever you feel like it. This is one of the most convenient options of dieting ever!

You are outside and cannot go into an eating joint, skip meal!

When you are hungry but do not have enough money, skip meal!

When you have a deadline in the office and you need to get things done quickly, skip meal and save time!

When you are late to the office, skip meal!

When you are too tired to cook or go out to eat, skip meal!

When you are not hungry but it is time to eat lunch or dinner, simply skip that meal!

This method is perfect to start your intermittent fasting journey. As there is ample flexibility of choosing when to eat and what to eat, you would not feel suffocated like most people do in a conventional diet! Starting intermittent fasting should not be troubling you in anyway.

Start with the method that suits you best. Do not go by the popular demand as your body is your own temple and you need to take care of it.

Benefits of Intermittent Fasting

Intermittent fasting has many benefits on the body and soul other than just losing weight. People largely take up intermittent fasting as a tool to lose weight faster without worrying too much about the food menu, but the diet has many disease fighting strengths.

Weight loss

People all over the world suffer from obesity, from the richest countries to the poor ones, you would find obesity being one of the crucial problems of all times. Intermittent fasting does not come with any high end food requirements that you need to go grocery shopping for. It is flexible to eat absolutely anything available in your local area. Because of its nature anyone can try this diet. Intermittent fasting reduces the hunger level and that eventually reduces belly fat. Without the 5:2 method of fasting, with intermittent fasting you do not have to worry about counting calories.

Insulin Resistance

Intermittent fasting can help you reduce the risk of type-2 diabetes as it reduces insulin resistance. It lowers blood sugar up to 3-6%. The insulin level goes up by 20-30%. This way intermittent fasting actually helps to combat type-2 diabetes.

Heart Diseases

Intermittent fasting has good impact on your overall heart functioning. It actually lowers what they call "bad cholesterol". It also reduces inflammatory markers, insulin resistance, blood triglycerides and blood sugar. All of these are working to keep your heart safe and risk free.

Brain Health

Intermittent fasting improves brain health. BDNF, the brain hormone is increased when one fasts. It is also said that it can be the cause of new nerve cell growth. Some research have shown that intermittent fasting plays a good role in combating Alzheimer's disease.

Inflammation

Various researches have shown that intermittent fasting can reduce inflammation markers. Inflammation markers lead to many chronic diseases. One can combat these chronic diseases with intermittent fasting.

Cancer

Cancer is a deadly disease and we're all well aware of how cancer patients end up. As there is no permanent cure for cancer, being cautious and prevention is always suggested. Intermittent fasting is considered as a solution to cancer prevention.

Anti-aging

A large market is surrounding anti-aging products today and from teenagers to old people, everyone is a consumer of anti-aging products. Intermittent fasting can organically help you be young and glowing all the time without wasting money on products. A study of intermittent fasting on rats was done and it showed that intermittent fasting helped them to live 30-80% longer.

Prevents over eating

During intermittent fasting, even a food lover who loves to eat would not overeat as the body would simply reject the extra food that is not required for the body. Overeating is a serious disease and it needs to stop in order to continue a normal healthy life. When you overeat, the feeling you get afterwards is not of enjoyment, rather you feel suffocated and lethargic. You should eat what you love but within limits. During intermittent fasting the body only intakes what it needs to move on with daily activities.

Decreases the junk food craving

We all have a craving for junk food and if you live close to a junk food joint or you cross a junk food joint on your way to office, then you are in trouble! The smell that comes out of the junk food joint is very seducing and hard for any food lover to resist. During intermittent fasting your junk food craving vanishes completely. You naturally want to stay away from it without even trying hard. The body knows what is good for it and therefore the body rejects that junk food craving.

Promotes a Healthy eating habit

Intermittent fasting unconsciously builds up a good healthy eating order in you. If you do intermittent fasting for at least 2 weeks, you would invariably build a good eating habit without you knowing it. Your body would train you when to munch on an apple instead of a candy bar! You would know by your-self, when to skip eating a cake and bite into a carrot stick to treat your sweet tooth!

Proper Sleeping habit

Intermittent fasting also contributes in building a good sleeping habit. When you fast, it is difficult to stay up late at night and staying up late at night is something that injures the health. Night time is for sleeping and when you stay up late, you get a nasty headache in the morning or you feel very dizzy all through the day. Intermittent fasting helps one to go to bed early and wake up early in the morning. This way you always get more things done and stay active.

What does Science say about Intermittent Fasting?

Intermittent fasting has been proven to be good for the health by doing several science backed researches on rats. The research has not been done officially on human, but only on rats. But many research results are found in rats are finding its similarity and authenticity seen in human behavior during the diet too. So even if you cannot rely on it by 100%, you can rely on the facts.

Intermittent fasting has been around since the ancient times. In the ancient times, the only source of cooking was open fire and people did not have so much readily available ingredients either. They had to search and hunt for food for days. They could not ensure 3 meals per day. They were trained to refrain from food by choice and by the situation. They survived well without food for days as their body was accustomed to it. They did not die out of hunger!

Many dietitians and fitness experts often suggest to eat like our ancestors did. The Paleolithic diet or the paleo diet is designed based on how our ancestors used to do it and it is one of the most popular diets of all time for weight loss and to remain fit. The intermittent fasting too is based on how our ancestor used to do it. It has many health benefits and with time people are starting to see the benefits as opposed to finding the cons.

The author of "Eat Stop Eat" Brad Pilon, who is an expert on the intermittent fasting method mentions while the popularity of the diet is increasing, with it the increasing fads surrounding it are also alarming. He is afraid that anything when becomes a fad, it loses it appeal sooner or later or in most case taken for the prime solution of everything. While intermittent fasting can work miraculously for weight loss and establishing a good eating habit, people should not take it to its extremity. For example, if you continue to do a 24 hours fast for the every other day, it may affect your health badly. Your body may not comprehend what you are trying to do and collapse. When you take things to extremity, often times a terrible accident is likely to occur.

In intermittent fasting where you get the open window to eat anything, many people take into account that they can stuff their face with junks food too. No diet can help you if you constantly crave for junk foods! The idea of intermittent fasting is to refrain from overeating and establishing a healthy eating habit. If you refrain from eating for 2 days straight and then eat as much junk food as possible for the next day, what good it can possibly bring? Nothing at all! That way you are only wasting your time.

Science proves that your brain needs brain food in order to function well. During intermittent fasting people usually try to feed themselves with food that works best for their tummy and makes them feel active. Most people during fasting consciously stay away from junk food because junk food gives you an instant sensation of gestation.

Research have found several health benefits of intermittent fasting like combating cancer, diabetes, increase in metabolism, developing a healthy eating habit, less lethargy, less obesity, combating inflammation etc.

The Food List

Every diet comes with a limited list of ingredients or a limited calorie scale to remain in but intermittent fasting neither has a calorie limit, unless you pick the 5:2 method of fasting, nor does it contain any list of ingredients that are allowed or forbidden. Only 5:2 method of intermittent fasting is limited to 500-600 calorie per day for 2 days.

Intermittent fasting allows you to eat anything you like and whenever you want it. There is no guideline, there is no restriction and there is no list!

But since this is a diet and you have started intermittent fasting for a reason, be it to lose weight, gain better lifespan, getting hold of your eating habit, combating diseases like cancer, type-2 diabetes or any other chronic diseases; eating in a healthy manner is always advised.

The fitness experts and other researchers would suggest to sticking to whole foods. This does not mean processed food is forbidden in intermittent fasting, but you need to know which food is good for your body and which are doing damage to your body and then decide whether or not you would want processed food in your menu!

Processed food is usually packed with added flavors, sugar, chemicals to keep it preserved for months. These added flavors, sugar and chemicals do harm to our body. They do taste good, but we need to weigh the taste with the damage it is indulging upon us. Once you made the call of cutting down processed food altogether from your menu, you would find many substitutes that are organic and has no added flavors or hidden chemicals in them. The worst thing these hidden chemicals do to our body is make us lethargic and fatty.

Switching to non-processed food may take a while, but once you get used to it, you will find it much easier to continue intermittent fasting.

For example, peanut butter sandwich is something we all love for breakfast, but the store bought peanut butter has many preservatives in them. You can simply make it at home with 3 ingredients. If you have a good food processor, it will take less than a minute to make peanut butter at home. The store bought one would also costs you more. Store bought ketchup is another example; this too can be made at home with very little ingredients and without harmful chemicals. Whatever food you are using every day for your menu, try to make it at home without any chemicals. This way you do not have to compromise on the taste and you will not damage your body either.

Processed food also contributes in gaining weight. So if you want to lose weight, this is another good reason to avoid processed food altogether. Sometimes the label on processed food is in their code names and people may not always know what code stands for what ingredient! This can be very tricky when you are a vegetarian or trying to avoid some food. For instance, Muslims do not eat pork and many foods contain pig fat in them. The ingredient list do not always say "pig fat" in it, rather it gives away a code specified for "pig fat". If you leave out processed food altogether, you will not have to worry about what code stands for what and accidentally eat something that you didn't want to swallow.

If losing weight is your main target when you started intermittent fasting, then of course you should only stick to a good balanced diet. A diet where every nutritious fruits and vegetables, meat, seafood and carbohydrate is present! You need to design your meal plan accordingly. Choose food that are good to increase energy level, lowers lethargy, and does not make you feel full. Intermittent fasting should leave you feeling light and good about yourself. If you feel full and blotted, then you are doing something wrong and you need to change your menu.

Lean protein is good to lose weight. Whole grains are also very essential for a balanced diet. Adding nuts, seafood, beans, fruits, seeds and vegetables should be added to your diet. Add dairy products too. They are good for your bone health and after the age of 30, people start to have bone decay and there is no better solution to this then eating lots of calcium dense food. If you cannot digest dairy products then switch to dairy substitutes like coconut milk, almond milk and cashew milk.

It is essential to combine your proteins with high fiber food to make your digestion process easier. As you are fasting, you may notice some changes in your digestion system and your bowel movement. This is natural as your eating pattern has changed. Do not be alarmed but be aware if some food is not working for you during intermittent fasting, you need to change it and adopt some new recipes with new ingredients. High fiber food is easy to digest but do not consume too much of it as it may cause diarrhea. So the eating pattern should be balanced.

Below is a list of a few ingredients that should be on the menu:

Water

As mentioned earlier, being hydrated is very essential during any diet and particularly on an intermittent fasting when you are refraining from food, it is crucial not to become dehydrated. You need to drink at least 8 glasses of water every day. Make a routine of drinking water every hour. You can also fill up a 2 liter water bottle with water and keep it somewhere you can see so you get a reminder of drinking water every time you look at it. Many people get gestational problems when they drink too much water. But the truth is if you do not drink enough water, your health would decay and your gestational problems would only increase. Dehydration also triggers many other problems in the human body like jaundice, fatigues, headache and lightheadedness. The last thing you would want in an intermittent fasting period is these health issues.

If you cannot drink water, try drinking fruit juices, vegetable juice, coconut water etc. Smoothies are another option but they have so much sweetening agents that only one glass of it should be enough for a day. If you are doing the 5:2 method of intermittent fasting, then leaving out the smoothie is recommended as it probably contains lots of calories.

Fish

Fish is a super brain food. It improves your cognition power. Intermittent fasting allows dizziness and sometimes messes with the power of your cognition. So eating lot of fish during intermittent fasting is a good idea. Fish is filled with Vitamin D and Omega 3 amino acid. There are not many foods where you can find Vitamin D. Vitamin D is very good for the heart, our skin and our growth. Fish has other healthy fats too. So to fill you up with lots of nutrition, fish is a great choice.

It can be any fish; there is no particular suggestion here. However, researches have shown fishes like dalmon and tuna have many benefits and are eaten throughout the world widely. Salmon and tuna can be found in cans too. If you live in a place where fresh salmon and tuna is not available, you can go for the canned ones, however; read the labels and see if any preservatives used in the can is particularly harmful for you or not.

Some people cannot eat fish as a whole, no matter if you make a fish curry, fish fry, fish soup or fish chowder, they simply cannot take the smell. In that case, try making **Fish Kebabs**. They taste very good and they do not have any smell of fish. If you do not tell someone the kebabs are made out of fish, they probably would not even guess it because of their delicious taste.

Apple

We know the saying,

"An apple a day keeps the doctor away".

It was said for a good reason. Apples contains many healthy nutrients like anti oxidant, mineral, magnesium, fiber etc. It gives you good digestion and provides you with healthy looking skin. You can eat an apple fresh or make a jam out of it and use it to make sandwiches. You can also make pancakes, other desserts using apple. An apple smoothie or juice is also quite delicious.

Banana

A banana is very high in calorie and some people rule out bananas during a weight loss diet. But a banana is very good for the health too. It keeps you energized for long and fills your tummy for a long time. So munching on junk food VS eating a healthy fruit, you need to decide which one you can go for!

Adding banana into your breakfast and smoothies is another option. Banana bread, banana cake is also very tasty and healthier option of baking. Whenever you have very ripe bananas or leftover bananas, make banana bread or banana cake, it will serve you good.

Seafood

Seafood like clam, squid, calamari and snail are very good for the health. They are very high in omega 3 and vitamin D. They are light in texture and require very little cooking and prepping time in the kitchen. They give you instant energy and keep you feeling active for about 6 hours. Try to add seafood to your menu every other day.

Fiber rich vegetables

Fiber is very essential for our body and when you are doing intermittent fasting, it can mess with your digestive system. Most people get constipation due to not getting enough liquid or fiber. The last thing you would want during intermittent fasting is getting constipated. To prevent constipation, relying on supplements, syrups or other herbal medicines is not always wise as most of these products have their side effects eventually. If you use them for a long period, your body will reject it and it may cause your constipation problem to get worse.

Finding a good solution for constipation is consuming good amount of high fiber food. Vegetables are a great source of high fiber. Vegetables like broccoli, cabbage, green beans, Brussels sprout, spinach, basil leaves, cauliflower, carrots etc are very fiber enriching. They can be cooked in various ways and to add variation to your menu, try out new recipes every now and then. The key to eating healthy is, keep on trying new things in the kitchen. One single cauliflower can be used in so many creative and tasty ways. It can be stir fried, it can be made into curry, it can be incorporated in omelet, it can be made a pizza crust, it can be a substitute for rice if you ground it, it can be baked as a whole etc. So if you try new recipes every now and then, the vegetable would taste differently and you will not feel bored of eating healthy food either.

Vegetable like broccoli is a super food. It has so many health benefits. Many people do not like the taste of broccoli or the smell of it. In that case, be creative in the kitchen and try making broccoli soup with mushroom, or make a stir fry broccoli and beef, baked broccoli with cheese on top tastes good too.

Avocado

Avocado is one such fruit that needs to be mentioned separately to emphasize its value! One avocado is enough to keep you going for 6 hours straight. You will not feel any hunger pangs or feel lightheaded afterward. It is filled with all the good nutrition. It is of course one of the highest calorie food, so you may wonder if you can eat it during a weight loss project, but research have shown it contains good protein, which is essential to burn body fat. It keeps you feeling full for a long time; therefore, you do not eat other junk food or snack for a long time. This way you are refraining from eating and it contributes in losing weight.

Avocado is considered to be a green gem. Avocado can be eaten by itself when it is perfectly ripen. You can make goat cheese and avocado salad, you can make avocado mash, avocado smoothie, and you can also make delicious dips with it. Adding avocado slices to your sandwiches also uplifts the sandwiches nutrition value.

Potatoes

Unlike other diets, the intermittent fasting has no restrictions or limitations on carbohydrates. So if you are a fan of potatoes, you are in luck. The fitness experts suggest, eating potatoes during intermittent fasting is good for you. It is the ultimate comfort food in any region and with the large productivity value, potatoes can be found anywhere in the world at any time of the year. It is rather cheap in price too. It is considered one of the most satiating foods too.

Many countries eat potatoes as their staple food. The countries that eat rice occasionally, makes mashed potato every day. So this shows how fulfilling the food is. Of course you cannot eat French fries, potato croutons, potato falafel, potato noodles, and potato chips and think that you are eating healthy food. You need to make proper dishes like mashed potatoes, potato soup, potato curry and baked potatoes etc. Store bought packed potato chips are one of the worse junk food you can eat, especially during a diet. It will make your belly blotted, give you bad gas problems, make you feel lethargic etc.

Legumes and Beans

While many diets avoid legumes and beans altogether due to their carbohydrate level, intermittent fasting encourages to enjoy a bowl of legume and beans packed chili every now and then. Legumes and beans are very good for your health. They contain low calorie and they keep you feeling full for a long time. A healthy diet should have a balance of every type of food and legume is one of them. Try to consume legumes and beans at least 3 times a week or more. It will still help you reduce body fat and give you a good eating pattern. Eating junk is always worse than eating calorie packed foods that are natural.

Legumes and beans can be added to so many recipes. Mexican chili is the first thing that may pop in all of our heads, but legumes and beans can be used for many other recipes like soups, stews, curries, even roasted. If you are craving for snacks, try roasting lentils, chickpeas, or beans with some salt and pepper. You have a good homemade snack ready within 10 minutes which has no artificial flavorings.

You can make amazing dips and guacamole using chickpeas. Chickpeas can be boiled and eaten with a pinch of salt and pepper and a drizzle of lemon juice. Lentil soup is one of the most comfort food ever during a winter dinner. So there are many good healthy options out there.

Oats

Oats is another super food which is one of the highest consumed breakfast items around the world. It is filled with all the good nutrition. Oats is highly fiber foods that help you digest well. It is a natural remedy for constipated people. It helps you combat many diseases as well.

Oats has a fallacy surrounding it that it is a boring food with no taste! This is so wrong and you would be surprised how many variations you can create with oats in the kitchen. To name a few, you can make oats porridge, oats pancake, oats pudding, oats burgers, oats stew, oats paella, oats tortillas etc. Oats is usually consumed with sweeteners but oats taste good when you make it savory too.

Nuts and Seeds

Nuts are a good choice to munch on during any diet. Nuts uphold numerous nutrition values. Nuts like cashew, almond, brazil nuts, peanuts, pistachios, walnuts, etc are considered very good for the health as they contain non saturated fat. Many think since nuts are high in fat, they may contribute in gaining weight. But non saturated fat actually helps reduce body fat and supplies you energy and keeps you active for a long time. The benefit of almond is very high. Soak it for 30 minutes, peel the skin off and munch on it. It will give you instant energy. Making a homemade nutty bar using these nuts is a good option for snacking. The store bought ones come with many added flavorings and sweetening agents that may trigger weight gain.

Seeds like pumpkin seeds, sunflower seeds are very good for the health too. Black cumin seeds are another super food you must incorporate in your every day like. They are extremely good for your overall health. It combats diabetes, cancer, gestational problems and inflammation. Many people just roast the seeds lightly and munch on them anytime they can. The smell and the flavor is rather strong, so if you think you cannot munch on it by itself because of the bitterness, you can add a spoon of honey or a date to accompany it. Adding natural sweetening agents will remove the bitter taste. You can also add black cumin seeds into stir fries and curries. People living in Asia, particularly in India, Bangladesh, Pakistan and Sri Lanka uses black cumin seeds in their curries and stir fries. Some even adds them to croutons and tortillas.

Dried Fruit

Dried fruits serve miraculously for providing instant energy. Dried fruits are also filled with nutrition. Dried fruits like dates, figs, plums, cherries, apricots etc are not harvested everywhere in the world, therefore, the need of making them dry came forth. They are pretty close to the fresh thing itself. If you soak the dried fruit for 1 hour or so in water or milk, it becomes softer and much tastier.

Dates and figs are filled with magnesium, potassium, calcium, folic acid, antioxidants, fat, and fiber. Can you think of many fruit that has all those macro nutrition value together? There are not many! So try to add dates and fig into your daily routine. Whenever you are craving for something sweet, bite into a date or a fig. They are high in calorie, so 2-4 per day is enough if you want to lose weight. When you are making a smoothie, instead of adding sugar, add 2 dates or 2 figs. It will make your smoothie thicker in texture and the taste would be mind blowing too.

The good thing about dried food is it can be easily stored at room temperature. It does not require keeping in the refrigerator. It will remain good for months if you keep it in a clean and dry place. Since they are dried, they can also be easily carried to your work place or wherever you are traveling.

Pro-biotic

Since this is an intermittent fasting diet, the chances are very high that you would feel hungry at times and the time before breaking your fast, you may feel the hunger pangs more than ever. This is natural but you need to feed your body with enough probiotics to survive the diet itself. If you faint or remain dizzy for the entire period, it will not do you any favors. It will in fact do damage to your body rather than doing good. So adding probiotic filled food in your menu is essential. Food like kraut, kefir is good for the health anyway and during intermittent fasting, they should be regularly consumed. Yogurt is good for digestion and skin too.

Berries

Berries are high in flavonoid. They work magic for your body and skin. You see how skin products and their commercial advertise always uses berries in them. It is done for a reason because berries contribute miraculously in keeping the skin flawless and young.

Berries like blueberry, strawberry, mulberry, raspberry etc all are very good for the health. They taste good too. You can eat 1 cup of any berry per day without worrying about the calories. Berries taste good anyway, so they can easily be eaten by itself. But you can incorporate them into pancakes, cakes, smoothies, juices and in some savory items too. Dried berries are also good.

Egg

Egg is a super food. Egg contains good amount of fat that is essential for our brain cells. Egg can be incorporated in our everyday breakfast, or in lunch or dinner in the form of an egg curry. Eggs are essential for baking items and if you love to bake then adding eggs into your everyday menu is not a problem at all. It will keep you energized for 4 hours straight. Intermittent fasting can take a load on the brain and your cognition power, so having brain food like egg is always good during these fastings.

Dairy

Dairy items are good for our bone health and cognition ability. If you can digest cow milk or goat milk well, then it is good but just in case if you cannot digest them, you can try yogurt, milk produced desserts that are low in calorie. You can also use substitute options like coconut milk, cashew milk, almond milk and soy milk etc. Often time people who cannot digest milk in its full form can digest milk based dishes without any hassle. Try making pudding, yogurt, and smoothies with milk and then consume it.

Poultry

As mentioned earlier, intermittent fasting does not restrict any food item and meat is something everyone loves but cannot consume well during a diet. With intermittent fasting, you can keep small portions of poultry in your everyday menu. White meat is considered good for health anyway. It does not cause any health related problems like red meat does. Chicken and duck are readily available in any part of the world. For turkey, you may need to search a bit because turkey is not raised everywhere in the world. Different types of birds can also be consumed with limited portion of serving. As your goal is to lose weight or live a healthier life, it is always important to portion control your meals.

Whole Grain

Whole grain is drawn out of many diets as they are filled with carbohydrates which trigger obesity. But a little bit of whole grain can actually help you reduce body fat. Whole grain keeps you energized and feeling full for long, which enables you to avoid eating more often. During fasting, you need food that would allow you to continue working at a good pace. Whole grain contributes to this criterion. Different studies have also shown that whole grain can actually rev your metabolism system. Rice it's one of the most popular grains out there. But there are many other options like farro, kamut, bulgur, millet, spelt, amaranth, and sorghum. It is time to step out of your comfort zone and try out these whole grains to see if they fit into your life well or not.

Staying Hydrated During Intermittent Fasting

Intermittent fasting has many methods and each one is designed differently. The most common thing any fitness experts or dietitians would tell their clients during any diet is to drink lots of liquid and to stay hydrated.

A dehydrated person is a mess and it causes many problems to the body. Sometimes even hospitalization takes place due to extreme case of dehydration. Intermittent fasting keeps you refrained from food for many hours and if you become dehydrated during the period, your body would get terribly damaged.

This is the reason staying hydrated is very crucial. You need to make sure you are consuming enough water throughout the day. Too much water can also damage the kidney, but too little water would do no good to your kidney and other organs too. So you need to find a proper balance here. You need to consume 8 glasses or 2 liter of water within 24 hours. A wise thing to do is keeping your bottles separate from other family members. That way you can detect how much water you have consumed so far and how far long you need to continue. A little more water would not hurt but it is best to hit the target and not miss it.

Many people cannot drink water and during a fast, consuming water becomes more difficult for them. In that case, switching to natural juices is the key to go. You can also try eating soups that are runny and broth like. Here you should avoid store bought juices and restaurant bought soups. Homemade things are always better as you know what ingredients you have put in and how much your body can handle. With store bought and restaurant made food, there is always a terror of consuming hidden chemicals that you are not aware of.

Simplifying Life

We are living in the 21st century and everything around us moves very fast. We are always on the go to get things done. There is no time to wait for anything or anyone. With our busy lives and a big list of chores to be done every day, if you can simplify your food intake and invest lesser time on it, would not that be great? There is hardly anyone who would not want to make the best use of the intermittent fasting process!

Intermittent fasting lets you simplify your life. It gives you enough opportunities to focus on other important things than just eating. People spend many hours in the kitchen every day, preparing food for hours. People also spend so much money on high quality restaurant style food and the end result is obesity. If you make some effort and understand how intermittent fasting works and try it yourself for 1 week or 2, you would discover how reassuring it is not to worry about the meals for 16 hours straight or longer.

The mother who cooks for her family knows the struggle of planning ahead of time what they would prepare the next day, how many dishes, portions, everything! They also need to go grocery shopping after they have made their menu plan. With intermittent fasting, the mother can relax for a while without starving her family.

Intermittent fasting allows one to refrain from food when they are in trouble and cannot reach food. The body gets trained and at the time of adverse situation, the body can actually sustain without food.

Who can do intermittent fasting?

When you read about intermittent fasting and its' numerous health benefits, you may wonder in your head if you could do it or not? You question yourself if there is a special criterion that you may not fulfill in order to do intermittent fasting! Interestingly anyone can do intermittent fasting. If you do not have any crucial health problems, then you can do intermittent fasting. You in order to know, for sure if your medical condition would not be hampered if you do intermittent fasting, check your doctor.

If you are in good shape, you have a sound health condition, then it does not matter if you are a man, woman or a child, you can do intermittent fasting.

Intermittent fasting for men

Intermittent fasting works different in men than in women. Men are biologically stronger and of different structure. Their body functions differently. What may affect a men's body may not affect at all a woman's.

Research has shown men have a better tolerance during fasting in comparison to women.

If you choose 5:2 method of intermittent fasting, then men should stick to 600 calories per day for 2 days of the week.

Intermittent fasting for women

As mentioned above, intermittent fasting or any diet has different impact on men and women. That is why many diets are more acceptable to men and many are not good enough for women. Intermittent fasting is good for both men and women but their body reacts differently during these fasting periods.

For example, a woman gets through menstruation every month and during that period they lose a lot of blood and energy. They feel very dizzy, lightheaded, irritated and they get many cramps and hunger pangs. Headache, belly ache body ache all of these come up for some during menstruation. To recover the loss of blood and energy, a woman needs proper and adequate food afterwards. So fasting takes a tol on their body and mind.

It is advised by dietitians and fitness experts to avoid fasting or being in a diet during their menstrual period. A woman can stick to 500 calorie bar when they are going for 5:2 method of fasting.

Intermittent fasting for Children

By reading the title you may wonder if the author has gone crazy that he is talking about fasting for children! Believe it or not fasting brings forth benefits for children too. Of course if your kid is mature enough mentally to do the fasting, then it will be beneficial for them.

Muslim kids fast for Ramadan, while they may not do the entire 30 days fast, but still they do a constant effort of fasting throughout the month of Ramadan. This shows that an average kid of 10 years without damaging their body and mind can fast and bring forth a better eating habit in their lives.

Of course you need to inspect if your kid is facing some problems during fasting. If they feel dehydrated, let them drink water and juices. If they ask to break their fast, let them do it immediately. You cannot force your kid to fast. If they make a constant effort on fasting, then do not oppose them and try to bend their decision. As there are no harms and benefits roven, then why not let them explore themselves if they like fasting or not!

Intermittent fasting During Pregnancy and Breastfeeding

Intermittent fasting is done by many women during pregnancy and while they are breastfeeding. Since intermittent fasting lets you refrain from eating for 16 hours and then opens up a window of eating for the next 8 hours; that 8 hours is enough to supply all your nutrition needs. Many women who have fasted during their pregnancy did not feel bad or brought any danger upon them. If you are on your 3rd trimester, the need of eating may increase and you may not feel as comfortable fasting as you did during your first and second trimester. In that case, skip fasting in the 3rd trimester. In the 3rd trimester your body also loses a lot of hemoglobin, so it may be best to refrain from fasting during 3rd trimester. You need to consume 2.5 liter of water in the eating window open period. If you can stay hydrated and consume high fiber, high protein packed food, then you would be good to go.

Breastfeeding moms too have fasted during their breastfeeding period and they did not notice any decrease in milk production. Research has proven these facts. So if you are breastfeeding, and still wish to do intermittent fasting, you can do it. Make sure to drink 2 liter of water in the 8 hours of open eating window period.

There are certain foods that cause to lactate. A breastfeeding mother should try to incorporate these food items in their everyday menu. Food like, oats, banana, mangoes, liquids, avocado, fenugreek seeds, black cumin seeds, milk, cheese, eggs, salmon, seafood, rich in iron food are very good to increase milk flow.

Intermittent fasting for Sportsman

A sportsman needs to be active and in a good health condition in order to perform well in the field. It does not matter if you are playing an outdoor sport or an indoor sport, your mind should always be focused and your health condition should be top notch. When you are feeling funny in the stomach or have a dizzy head, you would not be able to concentrate in your game. If you are playing a team game, then the pressure is even more. The agony of letting other people down on the team is crucial. So you need to maintain a well balanced diet all the time. Intermittent fasting is well balanced, it has many health benefits as mention in the earlier chapters. Intermittent fasting can be great for a sportsman as long as they maintain it well. As we know different sports requirements are different, and the method of fasting you are choosing should serve you well in your particular condition.

If you have a big match coming the next week, try to avoid extreme methods of fasting like 24 hours fast. Stick to 12:12 hours fast or 16:8 hours fast. An extreme fast method like 24 hours may make you feel lightheaded and it will affect your performance in the field.

Eat foods that are high in energy supply. Try not to eat something that is too tummy filling. We know intermittent fasting has no restrictions on food, but If you eat something that is too tummy filling, you would not be as active as you have liked in your performance.

A sportsman also needs to workout hard to remain fit and in shape. So make sure even during your intermittent fasting period, you are eating something high in protein before and after your workout. Nuts, dried fruits, smoothies, fresh fruits and vegetables are good option. Right before a workout session, make sure not to eat anything too heavy. It will make you lethargic and tired before you start your workout.

Intermittent fasting during long journey

We have mentioned it in the preceding chapters, how convenient it is for someone who did intermittent fasting in the past to go on a long journey and not worry about their food.

When you do for a vacation or a long journey by public transport, you cannot stop at any point, you need to go with the crowd. Food joints may not be available everywhere. Even if food joints are available, you may not like the menu. Bringing your own food in box is not always possible and it has a chance of getting rotten too. So at a time like this not eating is probably the best solution. Luckily for intermittent fasting dieters, they can refrain from eating on long journey by choice.

If you hit the eating window open situation during your long journey, you can munch on a good fruit or vegetable or nuts. Nuts and dried food are very good to supply energy and keep you active. Dried food and nuts can easily be taken any where as they are light weighted and they take up little space in your bag.

For someone who never skipped meals in their life would not be able to refrain from eating, even when there is no sufficient option available during a long journey. So, people who do intermittent fasting on a regular basis have an upper hand during long journeys.

Even if you do not eat anything during a long journey, it is essential to drink lots of water and other liquids to keep you hydrated. People often do this mistake of not drinking enough liquid during long journey because they are worried about urination. The vehicle you are traveling with will stop at an interval point and there you will find a proper washroom. So do not dehydrate yourself. The last thing you would want when you are traveling alone is getting sick or faint.

Intermittent fasting for Religious purposes

Intermittent fasting has been done for religious purposes in Islam, Christianity, Hinduism, Buddhism and Jedaism. It has been done in order to purify oneself. People from different religious perform the diet differently. Some choose to start their fast with the sunrise and break it off with the sundown. Some do it by the hours and some do it by counting the days. All of them have one thing in common, the need to please their creator. It is said to purify the body and the mind. It gives you a trans-like sensation and you also feel the pain a hungry person go through in their normal lives.

A homeless person or a broke person refrains from eating out of their need. They cannot simply provide for them 3 meals a day, therefore, they eat one meal per day or sometimes even cannot manage one meal. By doing intermittent fasting, you can feel the pain of a broken person and that way you refrain from wasting food. This teaching is taught by many religions as no religion endorses wasting food.

Intermittent Fasting before Exams

Right before an exam, the mind needs to be 100% focused. There is no loop holes here, your mind should be tension free and ready to give your best in the exam. Intermittent fasting can mess with your cognition ability. Therefore, it is best to avoid doing intermittent fasting before exams. It may affect your performance in the exam.

You can stop one week before the exam and start again with intermittent fasting after the exam. Even if you do decide to continue with intermittent fasting, make sure to get enough water and brain food in order to keep your cognition powder on point. Eating lots of nuts and good fat during these times are advised.

Intermittent Fasting and exercise

Most people take up intermittent fasting in order to lose weight. But refraining from food alone is not good enough to lose sufficient weight. You need to develop a good workout routine as well. You do not need to do hard cardio every day. A good option of exercise can be found in your everyday chores too. If you are a stay at home mother, your cleaning up the house, you doing the laundry, you going to grocery shopping can be your exercise. If you are active at whatever you are doing, you may not need to make extra time for exercise at all.

If you have to go to a place, say your office, instead of taking the bus or car or train, walk to the place if the distance is walk worthy. You need to be practical too, you cannot walk 5 miles to go to the office.

If you enjoy outdoors, try cycling, it will tone up every muscle in the body. Swimming is another great option.

Joining the gym is not always essential. You can find many sources of good exercise in your everyday activities at home or at office.

If it important to eat pre and after workout snack in order to be fit. Try not to drink or eat junk during workout sessions. Healthy homemade bars, nuts, fruits and juices are good options. Homemade smoothies are good too to boast your energy level.

There is no hard and fast rule on what type of exercise you should do during intermittent fasting and how often you do it. You should go with your body's condition. If you think a 10 minutes workout is fine for you, then stick to it. Not everyone's stamina is same. Some people burn calories without much effort and some need to work hard for it. You need to find your condition by yourself.

Possible Side Effects

Every rose has its thrones and like every diet, there are some drawbacks of intermittent fasting too. These drawbacks are not so much on the negative sides if you stay aware and be alert of the situation.

Intermittent fasting can only be harmful for you if you:

- Do not drink enough water and become dehydrated

- Take the diet to its extreme level and don't care how your body is reacting to it

- Only eat high calorie food

- Eat a lot of junk food

- Do not eat enough brain food or super food

- Do not maintain a good sleeping routine

- Do not do exercise at all

- Have major health issues and still continue the fasting

- Have diabetes and cannot refrain from food for long

- Are on medications

These are the few things you should check before you start the diet. If it is about health issues, like you have a disease or you are on medications, please do check with your doctor before you start the diet. It may give you trouble If you start without notifying your doctor.

Tips and Tricks for Nailing Intermittent Fasting

While doing intermittent fasting, there are certain tips you can follow in order to make the best out of this diet. You can also make intermittent fasting fun and anxiety free by doing simple tricks mentioned below.

Start the day with a glass of water

Drink 250ml of more water in empty stomach. This will help you boast your energy level and help you digest well all throughout the day. Do not drink zesty juice on empty stomach. It may give you bad gas and blotted belly.

Get as much liquid as possible

During intermittent fasting, it is crucial to get enough liquid to survive. You cannot get dehydrated; it will trigger other health problems.

Minimize Sugar intake

Try to minimize your sugar intake. Sugar can cause problem at empty stomach. Switch to sweet fruits to satisfy your sugar tooth. Fruits like fig, date, banana, dried grape can help you with this.

Avoid Oily food

Try and avoid oily food as much as possible. Oily foods mess with your cholesterol and give you bad gas problem too. Oily food during fasting is a bigger mistake.

Eat Yogurt

Try to add yogurt in your everyday menu. It will keep you energized and help you digest better.

Avoid oversleeping

Some people oversleep due to fasting, but oversleeping leads to cramps, feeling dizzy and more lethargic! Try to stick to a healthy sleeping pattern.

Avoid staying up late at night

Staying up late at night is deadly for health. It will give you terrible nausea in the morning, it will mess with your taste pallets, it will give you nasty headaches and it will make you a sloth eventually. Build a habit of sleeping early.

Wake up Early

Waking up early in the morning with the sunrise is considered very healthy. Go out for a walk and see the sunrise yourself. It has a healthy impact on the body and mind. It is great during fasting period as well.

Eat more super food

When you are making your meal plan for the week, make sure to incorporate as much super food as possible. It will make your intermittent fasting journey much healthier and easier.

Simplified cooking

Try not to over complicate recipes in the kitchen and invest hours on dishes. Try to meal prep ahead so you get enough time to rest during intermittent fasting. There is no point in working too hard in the kitchen during fasting period. Try to opt for simple recipes that take little preparation but taste good. Below you will find many recipes that are super easy and very quickly made.

FAQ on Intermittent Fasting

There are many conjecture that surround intermittent fasting. Here are a few of the most common questions asked about intermittent fasting and their answers.

- Is the diet safe?

Intermittent fasting has been done since ancient times. People used to do it for religious purposes and out of hunger. The former did it to impress their creator and purify themselves and the latter did it out of need. They remained healthy and very active for a long time. Today many research have also shown that it is very effective on weight loss. It has many other health benefits too.

- Would not I be dehydrated during intermittent fasting?

Chances are very high that you can be dehydrated in intermittent fasting if you do not make a conscious effort on drinking enough water and liquid throughout the fasting period. You need to keep count on how much water or liquid you have consumed. Make sure to fit the goal of 8 glasses at least. If you can drink more than 8 glasses; that is even better.

- Can intermittent fasting slow down my metabolism?

Intermittent fasting can actually boast your metabolism and help you reduce weight even with good amount of calorie intake.

- Should not I cut back on carbohydrate?

Intermittent fasting does not restrict you on any food, therefore, carbohydrate is also allowed. But make a conscious effort of eating minimum amount of carbohydrates every day.

- Should I count the calories?

Intermittent fasting lets you be free from the hassle of counting calories. Unless you are doing the 5:2 method of fasting, you do not need to count the calories at all. When you are doing the 5:2 method, you have 2 days to count the calories and keep it under 600 calories for men and 500 calories for women.

- Can I eat anything on the cheat days?

The diet technically does not restrict on any food, but it is not safe to eat anything during fasting as it will affect the body badly. If you eat too much fried food while fasting, it will give you a nasty gas problem. You should stick to healthy food of any kind. Junk food will not help you in any way.

- Can I stop at any time?

Intermittent fasting does not come with a plan where you need to follow it for a certain period of time. When you have successfully trained your body to refrain from food when you want, then you can do the fasting any time you want. Training you body to get accustomed to the new system would take few weeks. So during that period, stay consistent and patient.

- Does intermittent fasting really help in weight loss?

Intermittent fasting does reduce body fat miraculously and effortlessly. If you do it spontaneously for few weeks, you will see changes in your weight. Of course doing healthy exercise is a plus during the diet, especially when your aim is to lose weight.

Recipes

Breakfast

Healthy Veggie Juice

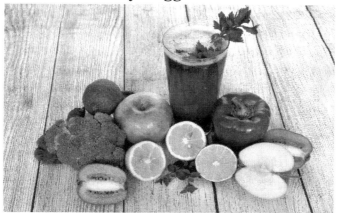

This is a power house juice
Preparation time: 10 min
Servings: 2
Ingredient:
- A handful of kale
- Fresh parsley
- 1 carrot, diced
- 1/3 cm of ginger root
- A pinch of sea salt
- 1 green chili, chopped
- A pinch of pepper

Direction:
- Add everything in a blender.
- Blend until you get smooth juice.
- Serve fresh.

Nutrition Facts
Calories: 122
Total Fat: 0.4g
Protein: 0.5g;
Total Carbs: 8g;

Plum and Flax Seeds Juice

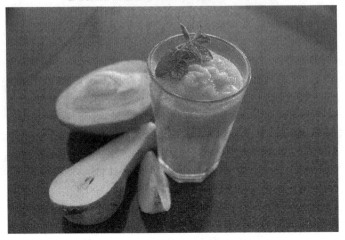

Plum is wonderful to eat and it is very beneficial for us too. Flax seeds on the other hand is very good for our digestion.

Preparation time: 5 minutes
Servings: 2

Ingredients:
- 2 plums, diced
- 2 small apples or pears, diced
- 2 cups of water choice
- 1-2 teaspoons of ground flax seeds

Directions
- Add all the ingredients in your food processor.
- Blend for 1 minute or until smooth.
- Serve.

Nutrition Facts
Calories: 122
Total Fat: 1.4g
Protein: 0.5g;
Total Carbs: 11g;

Blueberry pancakes

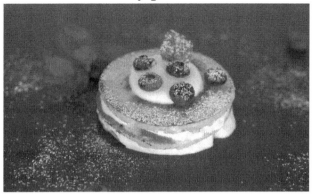

Preparation Time: 10 minutes
Cooking Time: 10 minutes
Servings: 2

Ingredients:
- 375g pancake mix
- 2 cups frozen blueberries
- 3 eggs, beaten
- 20g butter
- 1 lemon, zest and juice
- 1 cup water
- 1/2 cup icing sugar

Directions
- Whisk the eggs and combine with icing sugar.
- Add the pancake mix and water.
- Add the lemon zest, lemon juice and mix well.
- Add the blueberries and fold gently.
- Fry the pancakes golden brown in batches with butter.

Nutrition Facts
Calories: 342
Total Fat: 14g
Protein: 13g;
Total Carbs: 23g;

Green Pineapple

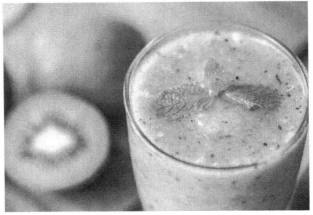

Pineapple combined with broccoli. This is something you must try at least once in your life.

Preparation time: 5 minutes
Servings: 1

Ingredients:
- 1/2 of a pineapple
- 1 broccoli, diced
- 1 cup water
- 1 long cucumber, diced
- A dash of salt
- 1 kiwi, diced

Directions
- Add kiwi, cucumber, pineapple, broccoli and water in a blender.
- Add the salt and blend until smooth.
- Serve.

Nutrition Facts
Calories: 251
Total Fat: 0.4g
Protein: 0.5g;
Total Carbs: 22g;

Orange Pineapple Chili

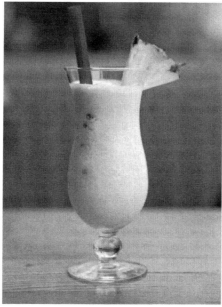

Pineapple juice tastes great but when you combine it with carrot, it is even better.

Preparation time: 5 minutes
Servings: 2

Ingredients:
- 1/2 of a pineapple, diced
- A pinch of sea salt
- 7 long carrots, diced
- ½ lime peeled
- 2 cups water
- ½ small chili

Directions
- Add the pineapple, carrot, chili, water, lime zest, and sea salt in a blender.
- Blend until smooth.
- Serve.

Nutrition Facts
Calories: 168
Total Fat: 1.4g
Protein: 2.5g;
Total Carbs: 22g;

Gingered Pear

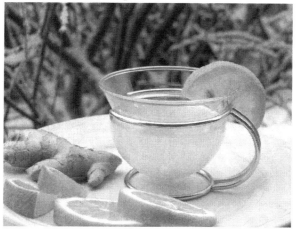

Have you paired pear with ginger? It is time to get creative in the kitchen.

Preparation time: 5 minutes
Servings: 1

Ingredients:
- 1 cup coconut water
- 2 pears, diced
- A dash of sea salt
- 5 celery stalks, diced
- 1 inch piece of fresh ginger root, minced

Directions
- Add everything in a blender.
- Blend until smooth.
- Serve.

Nutrition Facts
Calories: 142
Total Fat: 2.4g
Protein: 4.5g;
Total Carbs: 12g;

Low Carb Pancake Crepes

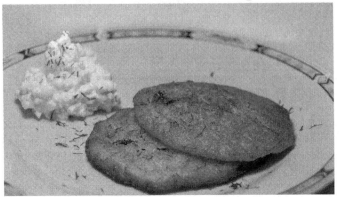

Preparation Time: 10 minutes
Cooking Time: 10 minutes
Servings: 2

Ingredients:
- 2 eggs, beaten
- 3 oz cream cheese, softened
- 1 tsp of cinnamon
- 1 tsp of almond butter
- 1 tbsp of sugar-free syrup

Directions
-
- Whisk the eggs in a bowl.
- Add the cream cheese, cinnamon, syrup and mix well.
- In a pan melt the butter and fry the pancakes golden brown.

Nutrition Facts
Calories: 342
Total Fat: 18g
Protein: 14g;
Total Carbs: 21g;

Pineapple Potassium Shake

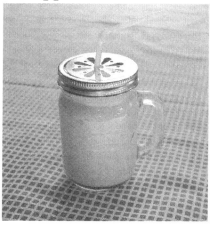

Pineapple is so good for the skin and body; it has many good nutrition values. Adding coconut water and lime juice gives this shake a good delicious uplift. Try to use fresh banana and pineapple juice. Adding frozen juices is also an option if you cannot find the fresh ones or they are out of season. There is no need to add any sugar in this shake!

Preparation Time: 5 minutes
Servings: 2

Ingredients:
- 1 cup pineapple juice
- 1 banana
- 1 cup coconut water
- 2-3 ice cubes
- 1 tbsp lime juice

Directions:
- Take the skin off the banana and dice it.
- Add to your blender.
- Add the fresh pineapple juice into the blender.
- Add the coconut water and lime juice.
- Blend for 1 minute and add the ice cubes.
- Blend for 30 seconds and serve cold.

Nutrition Facts
Calories: 187
Total Fat: 6.7g
Protein: 8g;
Total Carbs: 27g;

Avocado Coconut Smoothie

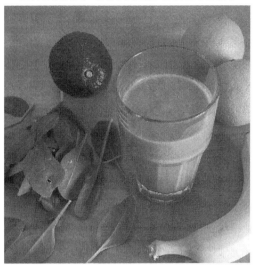

This is a powerhouse of nutrition! It contains banana, avocado, oranges and basil! What more could you want! You can add coconut milk, this is optional. You can use plain water instead of milk too. Adding honey gives it a better taste.

Preparation Time: 5 minutes
Servings: 2

Ingredients:
- 1/2 avocado
- 1 banana
- 1 cup ice
- Juice of 2 oranges
- 1 cup coconut milk
- ½ tsp orange zest
- 1 tbsp basil leaves
- honey to taste

Directions:
- Take the skin off the banana and avocado.
- Discard the pit of the avocado and dice it.
- Add it to the blender.

- Dice the banana and add to the blender.
- Add the basil leaves in the blender and blend for 30 seconds.
- Add the coconut milk, orange juice and orange zest.
- Add the honey and blend for 1 minute.
- Add the ice and blend for another minute.
- Serve cold.

Nutrition Facts
Calories: 424
Total Fat: 20g
Protein: 17g;
Total Carbs: 5g;

Low Fat Breakfast Cookies

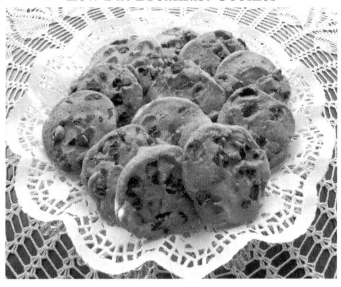

There is nothing like breakfast cookies! Cookies are many people's best friend and when you can make it healthy, you can eat it for breakfast without the hassle. This particular recipe has wheat flour, apple sauce, cranberries, etc all of these are very good for the health and gives us immense energy. Adding chocolate chips increases the taste and makes the cookie look better. You can substitute the apple sauce with grape or strawberry sauce too. You can use milk instead of water too.

Preparation Time: 20 minutes
Cooking Time: 12 minutes
Serves: 12 cookies

Ingredients
- ½ cup whole wheat flour
- 1 ½ cups rolled oats
- ½ cup chocolate chips
- ½ tsp baking soda
- 1 banana, mashed
- ½ cup light brown sugar
- ½ cup dried cranberries
- Salt to taste

- 1 ½ cup applesauce
- ½ cup all purpose flour
- 1 tsp vanilla
- 2 egg whites

Instructions
- Preheat your oven to 350 degree F.
- Take a baking sheet and spread parchment paper on it.
- Take a large mixing bowl.
- Shift the all purpose flour, wheat flour and salt together.
- In another bowl mash the bananas using a fork or a masher.
- Whish the egg white and mix with the banana.
- Add the vanilla, apple sauce and mix well.
- Add the apple sauce mixture to the flour mixture.
- Add some water to it to form dough.
- Add in the chocolate chips and cranberries and gently fold them in.
- The dough would be rather sticky; this will give your cookies a nice chewy texture.
- Use an ice cream scooper to scoop out the dough onto your baking sheet. You can also use a spoon if you do not have ice cream scooper.
- Make sure all the sizes are same.
- Bake in your preheated oven for about 12 to 15 minutes.
- Take out from the oven and let it cool down completely.
- Store it in a clean airtight jar.

Nutrition Facts
Calories: 260
Fat: 4.5 g
Carbs: 52.7g
Protein: 5.5 g

Flaxseed Smoothie with Spinach

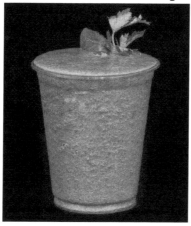

Flaxseed is very good for our digestion. Anyone who is suffering from constipation, flaxseeds can do wonders for them. This smoothie is a perfect boast lifter and a very good after workout smoothie. I add coriander leaves to this smoothie to make it more flavorful. You can also add mint to it.

Preparation Time: 5 minutes
Servings: 2

Ingredients:
- 1 Banana
- 2 tbsp Honey
- 1 tsp Flaxseed
- 1 Green Apple, cored
- 1/2 cup Grapes
- 1 cup Spinach
- 1 tsp Coconut Oil
- 1 tsp diced coriander
- 1 1/2 cups Coconut Water

Directions:
- Soak the flax seeds in water for 30 minutes.
- Discard the seeds of the grapes.
- Peel the apple and banana.

- Cord the apple and dice it. Add to the blender.
- Add the diced banana in the blender.
- Add the spinach, coriander leaves, grapes and coconut water.
- Blend for 1 minute.
- Add the coconut oil and honey and blend for 30 seconds.
- Add the flax seeds and fold them using a spoon.
- Serve cold.

Nutrition Facts
Calories: 469
Total Fat: 6.3g
Protein: 3.5g;
Total Carbs: 107g;

Healthiest Green Vitamin C Smoothie

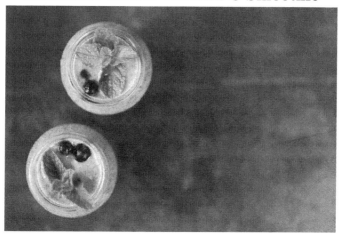

During summer time, you need lots of liquid in order to keep yourself hydrated. Drinking only water may seem boring, so to twist things up, try making juices and shakes using summer fruits like berries. Blueberries are very good for us and therefore I try to add blueberries in most of my smoothies. Blueberries and bananas balance the taste of kale here. Adding the lemon juice also increases the flavor.

Preparation Time: 5 minutes
Servings: 2

Ingredients:
- 1 cup blueberries
- 1 cup water
- 1 banana
- 4-5 Ice cubes
- 1 cup of Spinach
- Fresh mint
- 1 cup of Kale
- 2 tbsp lemon juice

Directions:
- Discard the banana and dice it.
- Add to the food processor.
- Add the blueberries, kale, spinach and mint.

- Add the lemon juice and water.
- Blend for about 1 minute.
- Add the ice cubes and blend for 1 minute.
- Serve cold.

Nutrition Facts
Calories: 250
Total Fat: 1.8g
Protein: 6g;
Total Carbs: 58g;

Low Carb Breakfast Waffles

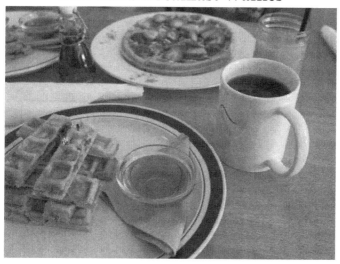

Waffles are widely eaten as a breakfast meal in many countries because they contains eggs, milk, flour, all of these contribute to boasting our energy level and gives us the ability to survive the day without full effort. If you have a waffle maker at home, you do not need to go out for breakfast anymore. This recipe is very easy and you can decorate it with any fruits, syrup or even cream. Adding fresh fruits makes it more fun and delicious. For me, a good waffle and a good cup of tea is all I need to start a working day. If you are allergic to gluten, you can use almond flour or coconut flour to this same recipe instead of all purpose flour.

Preparation Time: 10 minutes
Cooking Time: 15 minutes
Serves: 6

Ingredients
- 5 eggs, separated
- 3 tbsp full fat milk
- 2 tsp vanilla
- 1 tsp baking powder
- 4 tbsp all purpose flour
- 4 tbsp agave nectar
- 2 tbsp butter, melted

Instructions

- Melt the butter in a microwave and set aside for now.
- Ina mixing bowl add the egg whites. Use an electric beater to beat into fluffy firm egg white peaks.
- Take another mixing bowl and beat the egg yolks.
- Add the agave nectar and mix well.
- Shift together the flour and baking powder into the egg yolk mixture.
- Add in the melted butter, milk and vanilla. Mix well and make a smooth batter.
- Fold in the egg white mix into the milk mixture gently. Do not over mix at this point.
- Now heat the waffle iron and add one spoonful of the batter.
- Cook according to the direction of your waffle maker. Repeat the process with all the batter.
- Enjoy by adding fresh strawberries, agave nectar on top.

Orange Chocolate Chunk Cookies

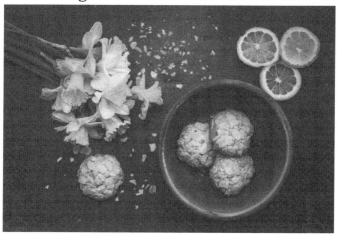

Cookies are one of the most versatile foods of all time! People can have it as a breakfast, a snack or even a dessert! If you make it at home with healthy ingredients, you can munch on cookies without any worry! This cookie is dedicated to oranges! It contains orange extract, orange zest and orange juice. The smell of it is wonderful.

Preparation Time: 20 minutes
Cooking Time: 10 minutes
Serves: 16 cookies

Ingredients
- 7 tablespoon butter
- 2 ounces unsweetened chocolate
- 2 eggs
- 1 teaspoon orange extract
- 1 tablespoon orange zest
- ¾ cup granulated Splenda
- ½ cup almond flakes
- 1 tablespoon orange juice
- 1 teaspoon vanilla extract
- ½ teaspoon baking soda
- 2 cups almond flour
- ½ teaspoon salt
- ¾ teaspoon baking powder

Directions:
- Shift the dry ingredients, almond flour, baking powder, salt, baking soda, and granulated sweetener in a mixing bowl.
- In a microwave safe bowl, add the butter and melt it.
- Grate the zest from the orange and squeeze out the juice.
- Use a knife to chop the chocolate into small chunks.
- Combine the melted butter, orange zest, orange juice, vanilla extract and orange extract.
- Beat the eggs and beat until fluffy.
- Add the dry ingredients gradually into the orange juice mixture.
- Add the beaten eggs and fold gently.
- Add the chocolate and add the almond flakes.
- Use a spoon to scoop the batter onto your baking paper.
- Bake in the oven for about 10 minutes.
- Take out of the oven and let it cool down completely before storing it in an airtight jar.

Nutrition Facts
Calories: 159
Total Fat: 14.3g
Protein: 4.37g;
Total Carbs: 2.26;

Buttery Date Pancakes

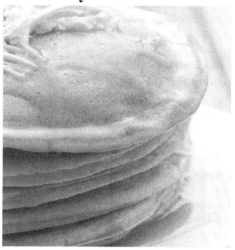

Pancakes are one of the most common breakfast items around the world! It is easy to make, it takes little preparation and cooking time and it is versatile. You can use the same recipe and add different fruits, vegetables and flavors to it. You can make it sweet, you can make it savory! You can make it using fresh fruits or frozen ones! The end results would be the safe, deliciousness! I have used the highly nutrition date here.

Preparation Time: 10 minutes
Cooking Time: 10 minutes
Serves: 3

Ingredients:
- 1/4 cup almond flour
- 3 eggs
- 1 teaspoon olive oil
- 6 dates, pitted
- 1 tablespoon almond butter
- 1 teaspoon vanilla extract
- 1/2 teaspoon ground cinnamon

Directions

- In a large mixing bowl, beat the eggs and make them fluffy.
- Wash the dates and cut them in half.
- Discard the seeds and mash them finely.
- Melt the almond butter and add to the eggs.
- Add the almond flour, olive oil and cinnamon.
- Mix well and add the vanilla extract.
- Mix into a smooth batter.
- Add the date paste and mix well.
- In a pan heat the butter over medium heat.
- Add the batter using a spoon and fry them golden brown from both sides.
- Repeat with all the batter.
- Serve with melted butter on top.

Nutrition Facts

Calories: 281
Total Fat: 20g
Protein: 10.5g;
Total Carbs: 4.5g;

Low Carb Pancake Crepes

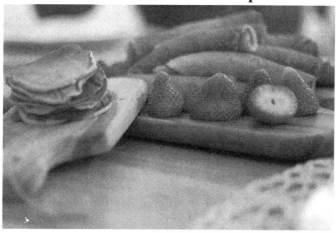

Crepes are one of the most fulfilling breakfast meal of all time. When you add cream cheese to it, it becomes extra healthy and super tasty too. Cream cheese has its own flavor and texture which makes the crepes rather soft and fluffy. I have added cinnamon and cardamom together; you can use only one of the spices or omit both of them and add vanilla extract to it. Use a nonstick pan while frying these crepes, it will be easier to fry them and lesser butter would be needed.

Preparation Time: 10 minutes
Cooking Time: 10 minutes
Serves: 2

Ingredients
- 3 ounces cream cheese
- 1 tsp ground cinnamon
- 1 tbsp honey
- 1 tsp ground cardamom
- 1 tsp butter
- 2 egg, beaten

Instructions
- In a bowl, whisk the eggs finely.
- In another bowl beat the cream cheese until it becomes soft.
- Add the egg mixture to the softened cream cheese and mix

well until there are no lumps left.

- Add cinnamon, cardamom, and honey to it. Mix well. The batter would be runnier than of pancake batter.
- In a pan add the butter and heat over medium heat.
- Use an ice cream scooper to add the batter, that way all the size of the crepes would be the same.
- Fry them golden brown on both sides.
- Repeat the process with the rest of the batter.
- Drizzle some honey on top and enjoy. You can add any fruit of your choice too.

Nutrition Facts
Calories: 241
Fat: 21.8 g
Carbs: 2.4g
Protein: 9.6 g

Quiche Lorraine

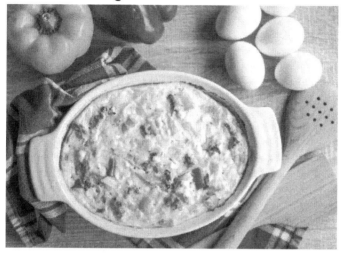

When you want a breakfast that would last you for 6 to 8 hours and you have the mindset of skipping lunch, this is the recipe you should go for without any worry! It is highly nutritious and healthy. It tastes great as it has the flavoring of nutmeg, pepper, and cheese. I have made it gluten free, that is why almond meal is used. You can use regular flour too if you want. You can add your choice of vegetables too. Tossing the vegetables for 3 minutes in oil will enhance the flavor.

Preparation Time: 10 minutes
Cooking Time: 1 hour
Serves: 6

Ingredients
- 2 cups almond meal
- 1 cup diced capsicum
- 1 cup shredded cheddar cheese
- Salt to taste
- Pepper to taste
- ½ cup melted butter
- 5 eggs
- 1 cup half and half
- Salt and pepper to taste

- A dash of nutmeg
- 1 tbsp mince garlic
- 1 cup mushroom
- 1 tbsp olive oil

Instructions
- Preheat your oven to 375 degree F.
- Use butter or oil to grease your baking dish.
- Whisk the eggs in a large mixing bowl.
- In a pan heat the olive oil.
- Fry the mushroom for 4 minutes. Take off the heat.
- Add in the capsicum, nutmeg, salt, half and half, pepper and cooked mushroom.
- Add the butter, garlic, almond meal, cheese, and mix well.
- Add to your prepared baking dish.
- Add some more cheese on top and bake in the oven for about 1 hour or so.
- Let it rest for 15 minutes before serving.

Nutrition Facts
Calories: 387
Fat: 29.6 g
Carbs: 11g
Protein: 22 g

Chia Seed Banana Blueberry Delight

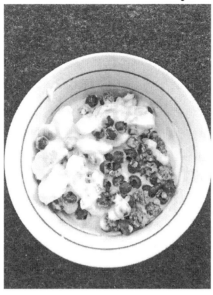

What if you can start your day with a delicious dessert like breakfast that tastes like a good restaurant quality dessert but does not cost you that much money or time to prepare it! On a plus side, it will leave you fully satisfied with your tummy and help you remain active all throughout the day. Chia seed is extremely good for our digestion system. When you pair it with banana, blueberry and yogurt, it becomes so enriching in texture and flavors. Adding nuts of your choice would bring crunchiness to the dish. I like to add dried date too in this recipes, it makes it tastier. The best part of this breakfast is there is no cooking required. If you have yogurt in the refrigerator, you can make this breakfast under 30 minutes.

Preparation Time: 30 minutes
Serves 2

Ingredients
- 1 cup yogurt
- ½ cup blueberries
- 1/2 tsp Salt
- 1/2 tsp Cinnamon
- 1 banana

- 1 tsp Vanilla Extract
- 1/4 cup Chia Seeds

Instructions
- Discard the skin of the banana.
- Cut into semi thick circles.
- You can mash them or keep them as whole if you like to bite into your fruits.
- Clean the blueberries properly and rinse well.
- Soak the chia seeds in water for 30 minutes or longer.
- Drain the chia seeds and transfer into a bowl.
- Add the yogurt and mix well.
- Add the salt, cinnamon and vanilla and mix again.
- Now fold in the bananas and blueberries gently.
- If you want add dried fruit or nuts, add it and then serve immediately.
- This is best served cold.

Nutrition Fats
Calories 260
Total Fat 26.6g
Total Carbohydrate 17.4g
Protein 4.1g

Egg Omelet

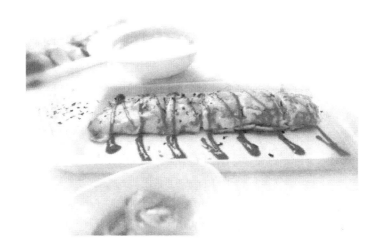

Omelet is one of the most basic things that people prepare with eggs around the world. Everyone loves it and as it takes only 5 minutes to prepare, it is one of the most convenient options out there too. I have used sausage, you can do it with leftover meat too. Adding mushrooms and other left-over vegetables would also work for making a good omelet. You can use more herbs to enhance the taste. Adding heavy cream to the eggs makes it more nutritious!

Preparation Time: 10 minutes
Cooking Time: 10 minutes
Serves: 2

Ingredients
- 1 cup cherry tomatoes
- 2 sausage, cooked
- 1 cup spinach
- ½ tsp oregano
- Salt to taste
- Pepper to taste
- 2 eggs
- 2 tbsp heavy cream
- 2 tbsp butter

Instructions

- Finely chop the cherry tomatoes.
- Cut off the stem of the spinach. Chop them finely.
- Crumble the sausage using hands.
- Melt the butter in a skillet over medium heat.
- Whisk the eggs with heavy cream in a bowl and add to the skillet.
- Top the egg with cherry tomatoes, spinach, oregano and sausage.
- Season using salt and pepper.
- Fold the omelet carefully.
- Serve with more oregano on top.

Nutrition Facts

Calories 289
Total Fat 53.9g
Total Carbohydrate 7.9g
Protein 19.3g

Savory Breakfast Muffins

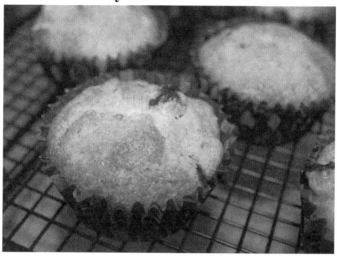

These muffins are not sweet but savory with spinach, cheese, chicken, onion etc. It tastes very good and for those who want to eat something spicy for their breakfast, can add some green chilies or red chili flakes to this recipe. I have used coconut flour and coconut milk for this recipe to make it gluten free. You can use regular milk and flour if you want. Almond flour and almond milk would work just fine too. This takes only 10 minutes to prepare and once you get them into the oven, you are free to do other chores in the house. You can use mushrooms instead of chicken in order to make it vegetarian friendly and omit the eggs with mashed potato.

Preparation Time: 10 minutes
Cooking Time: 35 minutes
Serves: 6

Ingredients
- 8 eggs
- 1 cup shredded cheese
- Salt and pepper to taste
- ½ tsp baking powder
- ¼ cup diced onion
- 2/3 cup coconut flour
- 1 ½ cup spinach

- ¼ cup full fat coconut milk
- 1 tbsp basil, chopped
- ½ cup cooked chicken, diced finely

Instructions
- Preheat the oven to 375 degree F.
- Use butter or oil to grease your muffin tray or you can use muffin paper liners.
- In a large mixing bowl, whish the eggs.
- Add in the coconut milk and mix again.
- Gradually shift in the coconut flour with baking powder salt.
- Add in the cooked chicken, onion, spinach, basil and combine well.
- Add the cheese and mix again.
- Pour the mixture onto your muffin liners.
- Bake in the preheated oven for about 25 minutes.
- Serve in room temperature.

Nutrition Facts
Calories 388
Total Fat 25.8g
Total Carbohydrate 8.6g
Protein 25.3g

Lunch

Shrimp Avocado Melt

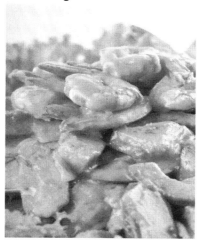

Avocado is a super food which contains many health values and with a little trick in the kitchen, it will taste super delicious too. Pick nicely ripe avocado, the ones that have not ripened yet would not taste as good in this recipe. This shrimp and Avocado recipe is from Mexican cuisine. The Mexican people would wrap it with tortilla, I am using lettuce leaves to wrap so it is on the healthier side. Adding nuts like almonds and cashew would uplift the taste and texture of the dish. It is a very creamy and cheesy dish, so make sure to burn all the calories with proper exercise. This serves both as a lunch of a heavy snack after workout.

Preparation Time: 10 minutes
Cooking Time: 5 minutes
Serves: 2

Ingredients
- 2 ounce shredded cheddar cheese
- 1 avocado, sliced
- 2 ounce shredded mozarella cheese
- 2 tbsp chopped chilies
- 1 pinch of garlic powder

- 2 tbsp butter
- 1 tbsp sesame oil
- 5 ounce cooked shrimp
- Salt and pepper to taste
- 1/3 cup roasted cashews
- 2 lettuce leaves

Instructions
- Melt the butter in a skillet.
- Add the sesame oil to it. Add the garlic and cook until it becomes golden.
- Add the cashew nuts, shrimp, chilies and toss for 1 minute.
- Add the cheese, salt and pepper and toss until the cheese melts.
- Transfer the mixture to a bowl.
- Add the avocado slices and mix well.
- Spread the mixture onto the lettuce leaves.
- Wrap them tightly and seal using a toothpick.
- Enjoy.

Nutrition Facts
Calories: 777
Fat: 63.9 g
Carbs: 23.7g
Protein: 36.1 g

Yellow Squash Soup

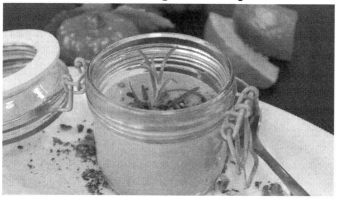

Squash is considered to be really good for the health. It is easy to digest and provides many health benefits. Squash soup during winter time is the perfect comfort food at any residence. This one is particularly special as it contains the goodness of almonds which add a lot of texture to the final dish and the heavy whipping cream and cheese make it quite nutritionally balanced. This dish can be your one meal for the entire day and you should be fine fasting the next day without any hassle.

Preparation Time: 10 minutes
Cooking Time: 45 minutes
Serves: 6

Ingredients
- 4 cups chopped yellow squash
- 1 tbsp olive oil
- 1 tsp butter
- 1 onion, chopped
- 2 eggs
- Salt and pepper to taste
- ½ cup heavy whipping cream
- 1 cup shredded cheese, divided
- 2 garlic cloves, mince
- 1/3 cup roasted chopped almonds

Instructions

- Preheat your oven to 400 degrees F.
- Add parchment paper onto a baking sheet.
- Arrange the squash cubes onto the baking sheet.
- Add some oil on top and season using salt.
- Bake in the oven for about 30 minutes.
- Let it cool down completely and then add to a blender. Blend into a smooth paste.
- In a pot whisk the eggs nicely.
- Add the squash, garlic, onion, butter, and salt and pepper.
- Cook for 5 minutes and add the whipping cream and cheese.
- Cook for only 3 minutes.
- Serve hot with roasted almonds on top.

Nutrition Facts

Calories: 228
Fat: 19.6 g
Carbs: 6.7g
Protein: 8.6 g

Meatball Soup

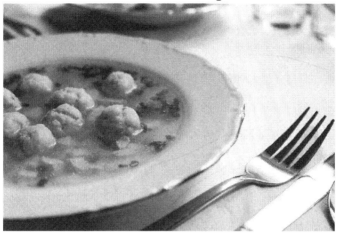

Soup is the ultimate comfort food in every season and during a winter dinner, it becomes heavenly. This particular soup is very rich in texture but gives you a light feeling even after relishing one bowl of it. The broth is clear and super flavorful because of adding the chicken stock, spring onions and fresh herbs. You can use turkey or chicken meat for this.

Preparation Time: 1 hour
Cooking Time: 25 minutes
Serves: 6

Ingredients
- 2 eggs
- 2 pounds ground chicken or turkey
- Salt to taste
- 1.2 cup soy sauce
- 4 cups chicken stock
- 2 garlic cloves, mince
- 1 tbsp butter
- 1 tsp ground ginger
- Fresh herbs of your choice
- Pepper to taste
- ½ cup sliced onion
- 1 tsp chopped spring onions

Instructions

- In a mixing bowl whisk the eggs finely.
- Add the ground chicken or turkey and mix well.
- Add the sliced onion, ground ginger, minced garlic and soy sauce.
- Mix well and use your hands to create meatballs.
- Cover the top of the bowl using a plastic wrap and add to the refrigerator.
- Keep it for marinating for 30 minutes or longer.
- Take a pot and add the chicken stock.
- Add the butter, spring onions, and season using salt and pepper.
- Now take out the meatballs and once the stock is at its boiling point, drop them carefully into the pot.
- Cover with lid and cook on medium heat for 10 minutes.
- Add the fresh herbs and take off the heat.
- Serve hot.

Nutrition Facts

Calories: 90
Fat: 6 g
Carbs: 0.8g
Protein: 7.8 g

Salmon with Spring onion and Sesame Seeds

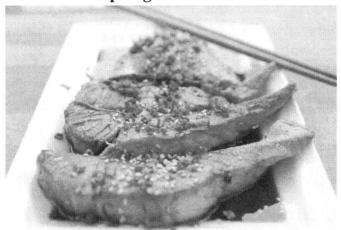

Salmon is one of the most consumed fish of all time around the world. Even areas where salmon is not found fresh, people eat it from the can because of its uncountable health benefits. The fact that picking out bones of salmon is rather easy than most other fishes makes it more popular. This is a simple Asian inspired salmon dish with soy and spring onions. You would be surprised to see how little ingredients can make such a flavorful dish.

Preparation Time: 10 minutes
Cooking Time: 20 minutes
Serves: 4

Ingredients
- 4 salmon fillets
- Salt and pepper to taste
- 1 tsp dried dill weed
- 1 tbsp soy sauce
- 2 tsp chopped spring onion
- 1 tsp sesame seeds
- 1 tsp onion powder
- 1 tsp sesame oil
- 2 tbsp butter

Instructions

- Debone the salmon fillets carefully.
- Season the fish fillets using salt, pepper, onion powder and dill weed.
- Let it marinate for 30 minutes.
- In a pan heat the sesame oil over medium heat.
- Fry the salmon fillets until they become slightly golden in color.
- Transfer onto a plate.
- Into the same pan, melt the butter.
- Add the sesame seeds and add the spring onion.
- Add the soy sauce and cook for 1 minute.
- Drizzle the sauce on top of the fillets.
- Serve hot.

Nutrition Facts

Calories: 262
Fat: 18.1 g
Carbs: 0.7g
Protein: 22.8 g

Cauliflower Leek Soup

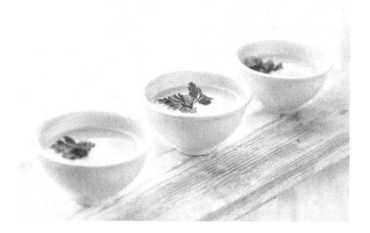

We have all heard about and perhaps tasted potato leek soup, now it is time to twist it up a little bit and try making cauliflower and leek soup. Cauliflower is very good for digestion and for health. The texture of this soup is very light and rich in flavor. Adding heavy cream makes the soup more thick. You can avoid the heavy cream if you want. The secret ingredient in this recipe is ginger; it helps our digestion process a lot and gives the soup a different taste.

Preparation Time: 10 minutes
Cooking Time: 1 hour
Serves: 8

Ingredients
- 3 leeks, diced
- 1 tsp thinly diced ginger
- 3 garlic cloves
- 8 cups vegetable broth
- 3 tbsp butter
- 2 tbsp olive oil
- 1 cauliflower heat, chopped
- Salt and pepper to taste
- 1 cup heavy cream

Instructions

- Cut off the stem of the leek and cauliflower. Wash them thoroughly.
- Chop them into small pieces.
- Add to a pressure cooker with broth.
- Cover and cook on high heat for 10 minutes.
- Use a hand blender to make the mixture perfectly smooth. If you do not have a hand blender, transfer the mixture into a food processor or a blender and then make it smooth.
- Now add some oil to a pot.
- Fry the garlic and ginger until they are slightly golden.
- Return the soup into the pot and mix well.
- Add the salt, pepper and heavy cream.
- Cook for another 10 minutes.
- Serve hot with fresh coriander on top. You can also add some fresh diced ginger on top too.

Nutrition Facts

Calories: 155
Fat: 13.1 g
Carbs: 8.3g
Protein: 2.4 g

Fish Carrot Potato Salad

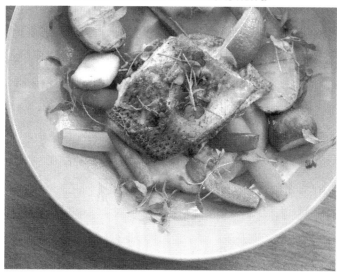

Salad is always good for the body and mind, and it gives you instant energy. This recipes uses fish to make a rather unique salad which is filled with fiber, vitamin D, omega 3, vitamin A and many more nutritious values. You can add more vegetables of your choice to this salad. Tossing the vegetables slightly over the heat makes it more flavorful. I have used tilapia fillet in the salad, you can add salmon, tuna, red snapper or any other fish in this recipes.

Preparation Time: 10 minutes
Cooking Time: 20 minutes
Serves: 2

Ingredients

- 1 fish fillet of your choice
- 2 carrots
- 6-10 green beans
- Fresh herbs of your choice
- 2-4 radishes
- 1 tbsp olive oil
- 2 small potatoes
- 2 tbsp butter
- 1 lemon

- 1 tbsp honey
- Salt to taste
- Pepper to taste

Instructions

- Discard the bones of the fish. Keep the skin on, it will add flavor to the salad.
- In a pan heat the oil over medium high heat.
- Add the fish and fry it until it becomes crisp.
- Transfer to a plate.
- Now peel the carrots, potatoes, radish and cut into thin long sticks.
- Cut the potato into wedges. Cut the lemon into wedges. Squeeze out 1 tsp of lemon juice out of them. Leave the rest for garnishing.
- In a skillet melt the butter over medium heat.
- Slowly fry the potatoes, carrots, green beans and radish.
- Assemble the vegetables, the fish onto a serving plate.
- Add lemon wedges, fresh herbs on top.
- Drizzle the honey and season the salad using salt and pepper.

Nutrition Facts

Calories: 152
Fat: 7.4 g
Carbs: 3.7g
Protein: 23.9 g

Dinner

Cheesy Broccoli Soup

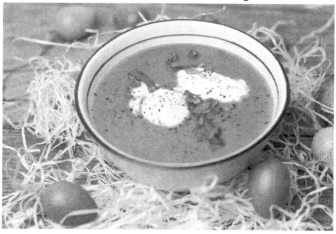

Broccoli is a super ingredient and but not everyone can enjoy the taste of it. Broccoli can be consumed more often if you try to make different dishes with it. I have added vegetable broth to it, you can use chicken or fish broth too. Adding cheese adds texture to the dish. Adding lemon juice gives the soup a zesty flavor.

Preparation Time: 10 minutes
Cooking Time: 30 minutes
Serves: 6

Ingredients
- 2 pounds broccoli, chopped
- Salt to taste
- 5 cups vegetable broth
- ¼ cup shredded cheddar cheese
- 1 tbsp olive oil
- ¼ cup lemon juice
- 2 garlic cloves, mince
- 1 white onion, chopped
- Pepper to taste

Instructions

- Heat the olive oil in a pan with medium heat.
- Fry the onion for 1 minute and then add the garlic. Fry until the garlic becomes golden in color.
- Toss in the broccoli and stir for 3 minutes.
- Pour in the vegetable broth.
- Add salt, pepper and mix well.
- Cook for 20 minutes or until your broccoli is perfectly cooked through.
- Take off the heat and let it cool down a bit.
- Add to a blender, and blend it until your soup is perfectly smooth.
- Transfer the soup into the pot again and heat it over medium heat.
- Add lemon juice, cheddar cheese and check if it needs more seasoning.
- Serve hot with more cheese on top.

Nutrition Facts

Calories: 97
Fat: 3.6 g
Carbs: 13.4g
Protein: 5 g

Beef Cabbage Stew

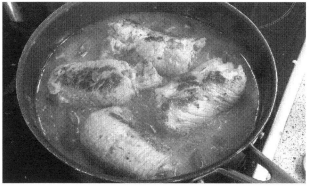

A stew is one of the most delicious dishes out there that does not require a master chef to create. This recipe is on medium difficulty level. With some dedication and time, you will be able to recreate it in the kitchen! The texture is rather amazing with tomatoes, cabbage, beef and the flavor is irresistible. You can use lettuce leaves for this recipes too. Some even use red cabbage leaves too. I have used beef stuffing, you can add chicken, shrimp, mushroom stuffing too. You can add cheese to the stuffing, it will add more flavors.

Preparation Time: 30 minutes
Cooking Time: 2 hours
Serves: 8

Ingredients
- 2 pounds beef stew meat
- 1 cube beef bouillon
- 8 ounce tomato sauce
- ¼ cup chopped celery
- 2 bay leaves
- 8 ounce plum tomatoes, chopped
- 1 1/3 cups hot chicken broth
- Salt and pepper to taste
- 1 cabbage
- 1 tsp Greek seasoning
- 4 onions, chopped

Instructions

- Cut off the stem of the cabbage. Separate the leaves carefully. Wash well and rinse off. Set aside for now.
- In a large pan, fry the beef over medium low heat for about 8 to 10 minutes or until you get a brown color.
- Into the pan, pour in 1/3 of the chicken broth.
- Add the beef bouillon, and mix well.
- Add the black pepper, salt and mix again.
- Add the lid and cook on medium low heat for about 1 hour.
- Take off the heat and transfer the mix into a bowl.
- Spread the cabbage leaves on a flat surface.
- Fill the middle using the beef mixture. Use generous portion of filling, it will give your stew a better taste.
- Wrap the cabbage leaves tightly. Use a kitchen thread to tie it. Finish it with the remaining leaves and filling.
- In a pot heat the oil over fry the onion for 1 minute.
- Add the remaining chicken broth.
- Add in the celery and tomato sauce and cook for another 10 minutes.
- Add the Greek seasonings, and mix well. Bring to boil and then carefully add the wrapped cabbage.
- Cover and cook for another 10 minutes.
- Serve hot.

Nutrition Facts

Calories: 372
Fat: 22.7 g
Carbs: 9g
Protein: 31.8 g

Quick Chili

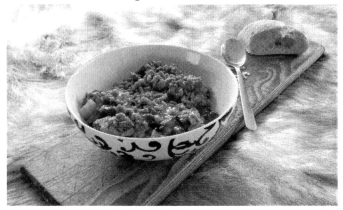

Chili is one of the most comforting foods throughout the year and people living in cold countries enjoy it more often. It can have any vegetables, any flavoring and it will still taste good. I have used pumpkin, you can add cauliflower, carrot or beetroot. I have used kidney beans, you can do it will lima beans or any other beans of your choice. It is best served with bread. You can also make it vegetarian friendly by omitting the beef.

Preparation Time: 10 minutes
Cooking Time: 1 hour
Serves: 4

Ingredients
- ½ pound lean ground beef
- 1 cup kidney beans
- 1 cup pumpkin, diced
- 2 cup water or stock
- 2 tablespoon hot pepper sauce
- 1 cup diced tomatoes
- 14 ounce tomato sauce
- 3 celery stalks, chopped
- 2 tablespoon oil
- ½ teaspoon chili powder
- ½ cup onion, chopped
- 6 ounce tomato paste

Directions
- In a pressure cooker, add the oil and heat over medium heat.
- Add the beef and fry until brown.
- Transfer the beef into a plate and add the onion.
- Fry until golden and then add the celery stalk, tomatoes and pumpkin.
- Add the tomato paste, hot pepper sauce and cook for 5 minutes.
- Add the bean and toss for 1 minute.
- Add the beef and pour in the stock or water.
- Cover with lid and cook on medium heat for 20 minutes.
- Serve hot with rice or bread. Some even eat it as it is.

Nutrition Facts
Calories: 248
Total Fat: 10g
Protein: 18g;
Total Carbs: 28.4g;

Fried Whole Tilapia

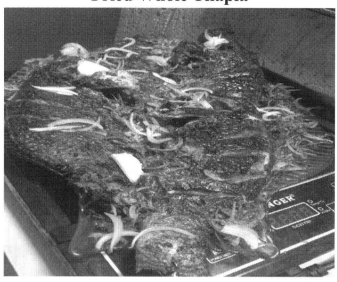

Whenever I am making whole fish, I always worry about cutting and cleaning it, because if you cut it badly, it will show on the plate after serving it. This is a good choice of fish dish when you have guests coming into the house. The marinated onion fries tastes heavenly. This dish will give you the feeling of eating junk food at home. This type of dish is something you should treat yourself with only occasionally. After you have lost a few pounds, you can celebrate with this type of dish. Do not eat it every other day, it may give you bad gas problems.

Preparation Time: 10 minutes
Cooking Time: 25 minutes
Serves: 2

Ingredients
- 10 ounce tilapia
- 2 tbsp oil
- 5 garlic cloves, mince
- 4 large onion ,chopped
- 2 tbsp red chili powder
- 1 tsp turmeric powder
- 1 tsp cumin powder

- 1 tsp coriander powder
- Salt to taste
- Black pepper to taste
- 2 tbsp soy sauce
- 2 tbsp fish sauce

Instructions

- Take the tilapia fish and clean it well without taking off the skin. You need to fry it whole, so you have to be careful about cleaning the gut inside.
- Cut few slits on the skin so the seasoning gets inside well.
- Marinate the fish with fish sauce, soy sauce, red chili powder, cumin powder, turmeric powder, coriander powder, salt and pepper.
- Coat half of the onions in the same mixture too.
- Let them marinate for 1 hour.
- In a skillet heat the oil. Fry the fish for 8 minutes on each side.
- Transfer the fish into serving plate.
- Fry the marinated onions until they become crispy.
- Add the remaining raw onions on top and serve hot.

Nutrition Facts

Calories: 368
Fat: 30.1 g
Carbs: 9.2g
Protein: 16.6 g

African Chicken Curry

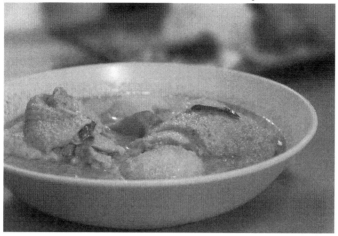

When you want something heavy, like a curry, try this recipe. It is African style curry with chicken. You can do the same recipe using beef or lamb. It will taste just as good, but in case of red meat, it may take 20 to 30 minutes extra to make the meat tender enough. Keeping the skin on the chicken adds a lot of flavor to the curry. Adding coconut milk also brings in more texture and thickness.

Preparation Time: 10 minutes
Cooking Time: 30 minutes
Serves: 4

Ingredients

- 1 pound whole chicken
- 1/2 onion
- 1/2 cup coconut milk
- 1/2 bay leaf
- 1-1/2 teaspoon olive oil
- 1/2 cup peeled tomatoes
- 1 teaspoon curry powder
- 1/8 teaspoon salt
- 1/2 lemon, juiced
- 1 clove garlic

Directions
- Keep the skin of the chicken.
- Cut your chicken into 8 pieces. It looks good when you keep the size not too small or not too big.
- Discard the skin of the onion and garlic and mince the garlic and dice the onion.
- Cut the tomato wedges.
- Now in a pot add the olive oil and heat over medium heat.
- Add the garlic and fry until it becomes brown.
- Add the diced onion and caramelize it.
- Add the bay leaf, and chicken pieces.
- Fry the chicken pieces until they are golden.
- Add the curry powder, coconut milk and salt.
- Cover and cook for 10 minutes on high heat.
- Turn the heat to medium low and add the lemon juice.
- Add the tomato wedges and the coconut milk.
- Cook for another 10 minutes.
- Serve hot with rice or tortilla.

Nutrition Facts
Calories: 354
Total Fat: 10g
Protein: 18g;
Total Carbs: 17g;

Yummy Garlic Chicken Livers

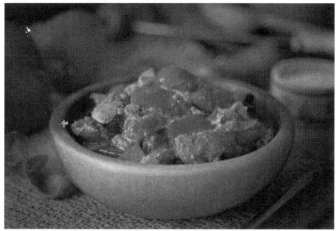

Chicken liver is something people usually do not eat throughout the world. Some people love it and some people are doubtful about the taste and the cooking method. Liver is a great source of iron and if you can cook it properly, it will taste heavenly. Cooking this dish is not too hard, follow the instructions carefully and you will be able to put it off. I have added tomatoes; you can add capsicum here too. You can use this same recipe for making cow liver too, in that case; increase the cooking time by 20 minutes.

Preparation Time: 10 minutes
Cooking Time: 30 minutes
Serves: 2

Ingredients

- ½ pound chicken liver
- 2 teaspoon lime juice
- 6 garlic cloves, mince
- ½ teaspoon salt
- 1 tbsp ginger garlic paste
- 1 cup diced onion
- 1 tbsp red chili powder
- 1 tsp cumin
- 1 tsp coriander powder
- Black pepper to taste

- 1 cardamom
- 2 tomatoes
- 1 cinnamon stick
- 1 bay leaf
- 4 tablespoon olive oil

Directions
- In a large pan, heat your oil over high heat.
- Add the garlic and fry them golden brown.
- Add onion and fry until they become caramelized.
- Turn the heat to medium and add the bay leaf, cinnamon stick, cardamom and toss for 30 seconds.
- Add the ginger garlic paste and 1 tbsp water. Adding water prevents burning.
- Add the coriander powder, black pepper, salt, cumin, and red chili powder.
- Cover and cook on low heat for 3 minutes.
- Add the livers and cook on medium heat for 15 minutes.
- Add the tomatoes and cook for another 5 minutes.
- Check the seasoning, add more salt if needed.
- Serve hot with tortilla.

Nutrition Facts
Calories: 174
Total Fat: 9g
Protein: 18g;
Total Carbs: 2.4g

Healthy Chickpea Burger

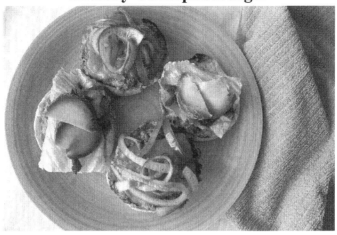

This is absolutely mind blowing in terms of taste and health value. You can get creative and add more toppings of your choice. There is no hard and fast rule.

Preparation Time: 15 minutes
Cooking Time: 10 minutes
Serves: 2

Ingredients:
- 1 cup chickpeas, boiled
- 1 tbsp tomato puree
- 1 tsp soy sauce
- A pinch of paprika
- A pinch of white pepper
- 1 onion, diced
- Salt to taste
- 2 lettuce leaves
- ½ cup bell pepper, sliced
- 1 tsp olive oil
- 1 avocado, sliced
- 2 Burger buns to serve

Instructions:
- Mash the chickpeas and combine with bell pepper, salt, pepper, paprika, soy sauce and tomato puree.
- Use your hands to make patties.
- Fry the patties golden brown with oil.
- Assemble the burgers with lettuce, onion, avocado and enjoy.

Nutrition Facts
Calories: 254
Total Fat: 12g
Protein: 9g;
Total Carbs: 7.8g;

Croutons Cabbage and Egg Salad

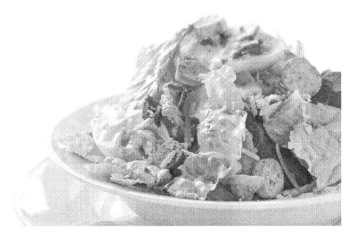

This is one of the healthiest salads I have ever tried. It has protein, carb, fat and fiber.

Preparation Time: 15 minutes
Serves: 2

Ingredients:
- 2 eggs, boiled
- 6-8 croutons
- 1 cup cabbage, cubed
- ½ cup lettuce, torn
- 2 tbsp cheddar cheese
- ½ cup Greek Yogurt
- Salt to taste
- White pepper to taste
- Any nuts of your choice, chopped

Instructions:
- Cut the eggs into pieces.
- Combine the yogurt, pepper, cheddar cheese, in a bowl.
- Add the eggs, croutons, cabbage, lettuce, and nuts.
- Serve.

Nutrition Facts
Calories: 264
Total Fat: 14g
Protein: 14g;
Total Carbs: 8g;

Creamy Chicken Soup

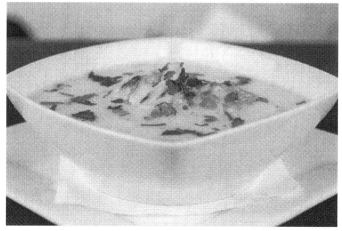

This is the perfect comfort food during winter time.

Preparation Time: 15 minutes
Cooking Time: 30 minutes
Serves: 4

Ingredients:
- 1 egg, beaten
- 1 cup chicken breast, diced
- 1 tsp butter
- 1 tsp white pepper
- 1 cup milk
- Salt to taste
- 1 cube of chicken stock
- Fresh coriander
- 1 green chili
- 1 sprig of lemongrass
- 1 tsp lemon juice

Instructions:
- In a pressure cooker, add everything together and mix well.
- Cover and cook on low heat for 10 minutes.
- Stir once and again cook on medium high heat for 10 minutes.
- Serve hot.

Nutrition Facts
Calories: 364
Total Fat: 14g
Protein: 19g;
Total Carbs: 11g;

Snack

Rosemary and Sea Salt Zucchini Chips

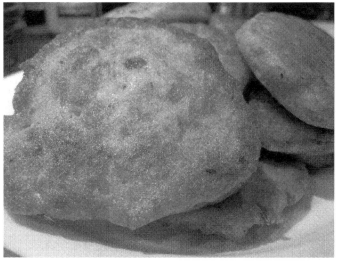

Zucchini is very good and high in fiber. Turning zucchini into a snack that tastes good is not a challenge when you have such a easy recipe like this. It can be prepared within 10 minutes. Adding herbs like rosemary enhances the taste. You can add any herb of your choice.

Preparation Time: 10 minutes
Cooking Time: 5 minutes
Serves: 2

Ingredients
- 2 tsp dried rosemary
- 2 large zucchini
- 1 tsp sea salt
- 1 tbsp coconut oil, melted
- 1 cup chickpea flour
- Water as needed

Directions
- Take the zucchinis and wash them thoroughly.
- Peel then using a knife or peeler.
- Cut into thin sliced. The slice should be thin enough to see your fingers through the other side. The thinner you cut, the better it will taste.
- Combine the chickpea flour with water and salt.
- Add small portion of water at a time and keep mixing until you get a semi thick batter. It the batter is too thick, it will taste bad, but if it is too thin and runny then it will not stick to your zucchini slices.
- Heat the oil in a skillet over medium high heat.
- Add the rosemary into the batter and mix well.
- Dip each zucchini slice into the batter and fry into the hot water until it becomes golden brown.
- Make sure to fry in batches to get the best result.
- Serve hot with a dipping sauce of your choice.

Nutrition Facts
Calories: 92g
Total Fat: 4g
Protein: 0.5g;
Total Carbs: 17g;
Dietary Fiber: 4.6g; Sugars: 0.2g

Paleo Power Balls

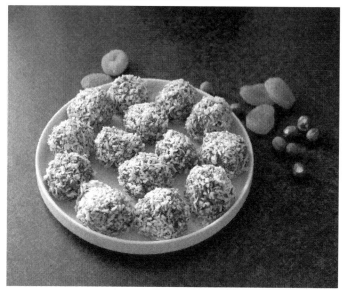

Have you ever eaten power balls using plum, nuts, dates and combine it with a super food like sweet potato? This sounds bizarre but tastes rather delicious. The power ball is very powerful in terms of boasting your energy level. It can be eaten as a heavy after workout snack or as dessert too. Adding date is very essential in this recipe, you cannot substitute it. You can add any nuts and dried fruit of your choice.

Preparation Time: 20 minutes
Cooking Time: 10 minutes
Serves: 4

Ingredients:
- 1 sweet potato
- 4-6 dried plum
- 2 tbsp chopped nuts of your choice
- 1 cup shredded coconut
- 3 egg yolks
- 2 teaspoon honey
- 3 Tablespoon coconut flour
- 4 Tablespoon melted Coconut Oil
- 1 teaspoon vanilla powder

- 2 cups almond meal
- 3 teaspoon baking powder

Directions

- Peel the sweet potato and cut it into wedges.
- Add the sweet potato in a pot. Pour enough water to cover the sweet potatoes.
- Cook until the sweet potatoes are boiled. Do not over boil it.
- Drain well and rinse the water completely.
- Mash using a fork or a masher.
- In a mixing bowl add the almond meal, coconut flour, dried plum, shredded coconut, vanilla powder, and baking powder.
- Add the sweet potato mash and mix well.
- Add the egg yolks and honey.
- Knead well into a sticky dough.
- Add some oil into your hands and create small balls using the mixture.
- Arrange desiccated coconut onto a plate.
- Roll the balls onto the coconut and let them come to room temperature before serving them.

Nutrition Facts

Calories: 280
Total Fat: 34g
Protein: 18g;
Total Carbs: 20g;

Easy Kale Chips

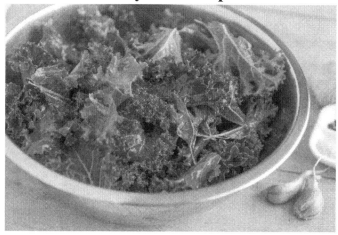

Kale is a super green food that is filled with many nutritious components. This recipe can be made both by deep frying them or baking them into the oven. The healthier version is definitely when you use less oil in the oven. This serves as a great snack!

Preparation Time: 10 minutes
Cooking Time: 10 minutes
Serves: 2

Ingredients
- 2 tbsp olive oil
- 1 bunch of kale
- Sea salt to taste

Directions
- Remove the stem off the kale.
- Wash them carefully few times until they are ready to use.
- Rinse them well and add salt to season it.
- If you are baking them, place a parchment paper onto your baking sheet.
- Preheat the oven to 170 degrees F.
- Arrange the kale pieces onto the baking sheet.
- Add the oil on top.
- Bake in the preheated oven for about 20 minutes.

- Let them cool down for 5 minutes before eating them.
- IF you are frying them, heat the oil in a pan and fry them for 5 minutes only.
- Serve warm.

Nutrition Facts
Calories: 140
Total Fat: 1.2g
Protein: 0.0g;
Total Carbs: 5.3g

Baked Cinnamon Apple Chips

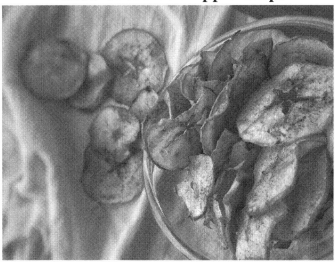

We know apple is a super food and eating it as a whole is not always fun. If you want to keep an apple in your regular meals, you need to try different recipes like this. It tastes rather good and it gives you the feeling of eating junk food without giving you any bad side effects of junk food! The same recipe can be tried with pears too. Here using oil is totally optional, you can omit it if you like.

Preparation Time: 10 minutes
Cooking Time: 30 minutes
Serves: 2

Ingredients
- 1 tsp cinnamon powder
- A pinch of star anise powder
- 2 red apples
- 1 tbsp olive oil

Directions
- Preheat the oven to 180 degrees F.
- Take your apples and wash them well.
- Use a peeler to discard the skin.
- Cut them into thin circles using a knife.

- Remove the seeds carefully.
- Add parchment paper onto your baking sheet.
- Arrange the apple slices.
- Sprinkle the cinnamon powder, star anise powder and add the oil.
- Bake in the oven for 30 minutes.
- Let them cool down completely and then eat it. You can store them in a tight jar for 1 week too.

Nutrition Facts
Calories: 127g
Total Fat: 11g
Protein: 8g;
Total Carbs: 18g

Thai Spiced Turkey Patties

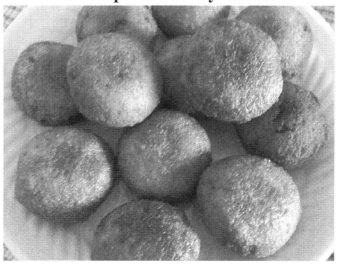

When you know it is too late for lunch but your stomach is craving something more than nuts and fruits, then turning to these fabulous turkey patties snack is a great idea! They are not at all complicated to make. They can be frozen for up to 3 months. So you make a big batch and enjoy these treats for a long time.

Preparation Time: 30 minutes
Cooking Time: 5 minutes
Serves: 4

Ingredients
- 2 garlic cloves, crushed
- 800g ground turkey
- Zest and juice 1 lime
- 2 tbsp olive oil
- 500g pack mixed peppers
- 4 nests medium zucchini noodles, cooked
- 1 lemongrass stalk, finely chopped
- 2 tbsp coriander, chopped
- 6 tbsp tomato sauce
- 3 red chili, chopped

Directions

- Take a large mixing bowl.
- Add the ground turkey, crushed garlic, lime juice, lime zest, coriander, lemongrass stalk, peppers, and zucchini noodles.
- Add salt to taste.
- Mix using your hands and make sure everything is well coated.
- Create flat little patties in the size you want.
- In a skillet heat the oil over medium high heat.
- Fry the patties in batches until they become golden brown.
- If you want to freeze them, make sure to pack them well using plastic wrapper.
- Serve the patties warm.

Nutrition Facts

Calories: 454
Total Fat: 24g
Protein: 29g;
Total Carbs: 19g;

Healthy Salmon Burgers

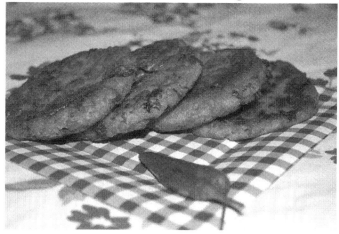

Fried food and patties does not always have to be unhealthy for you! When you use ingredients like salmon and use very little oil, occasionally feeding yourself these is not a bad idea. They will give you energy and a treat to your taste buds. Combine it with yogurt and your snacking experience would get uplifted. This can be a good after workout snack.

Preparation Time: 10 minutes
Cooking Time: 10 minutes
Serves: 6

Ingredients
- 2 salmon fillets
- 2 eggs
- 1/2 cup chopped onions
- 1 tbsp mayonnaise
- 1 cup gluten-free bread crumbs
- 2 tsp lemon juice
- 1/4 tsp garlic salt
- 1 tbsp chopped fresh parsley
- 3 tbsp olive oil

Directions

- Season the salmon using salt and pepper.
- In a skillet add ½ tbsp of oil and heat it over medium heat.
- Fry the salmon for 2 minutes on both sides.
- Let it cool down completely.
- Remove them bones and mash it finely.
- In a bowl transfer the salmon. Add the onion, garlic salt, parsley, bread crumbs, mayo and eggs.
- Mix well and create burger patties using your hands.
- Let it refrigerate for 30 minutes.
- In a skillet heat the remaining oil.
- Once the oil is hot enough fry the patties golden brown.
- Make sure to fry in batches.
- Serve warm.

Nutrition Facts

Calories: 254
Total Fat: 20g
Protein: 15g;
Total Carbs: 8g;

7 day Meal plan

Here is a rough meal plan for the first week of fasting. You can of course twist it, omit certain recipes and add your own unique touches. Intermittent fasting has no hard and fast rules on anything as long as you are eating healthy and what is good for you.

	Day1	Day2	Day3	Day4	Day5	Day6	Day7
Breakfast	Quiche Lorraine	Avocado Coconut Smoothie	Low Carb Breakfast Waffles	Buttery Date Pancakes	Avocado Coconut Smoothie	Low Carb Breakfast Waffles	Buttery Date Pancakes
Lunch	Quick Chili	Beef Cabbage Stew	Fish Carrot Potato Salad	Quick Chili	Cheesy Broccoli Soup	Beef Cabbage Stew	Yellow Squash Soup
Dinner	Fish Carrot Potato Salad	Quick Chili	Cheesy Broccoli Soup	Beef Cabbage Stew	Yellow Squash Soup	Quick Chili	Fish Carrot Potato Salad
Snack/Dessert	Paleo Power Balls	Healthy Salmon Burgers	Paleo Power Balls	Baked Cinnamon Apple Chips	Rosemary and Sea Salt Zucchini Chips	Healthy Salmon Burgers	Paleo Power Balls

Conclusion

Intermittent fasting comes with many benefits and the best part is there are no restrictions on what and when you can eat! Many people take up this diet only to live a better life with a healthy eating habit.

Of course in addition you would get a fantastic body and skin. The feeling that intermittent fasting leaves you with is amazing.

This book has many things where a newbie trying intermittent fasting would feel clear that this is what they need to do and achieve. The diet comes with freedom. Freedom is what makes us happy even when we are in a diet.

Keep the important things in mind while you are in the diet, like being hydrated, keeping away from too much junk food, doing moderate exercise etc.

If you have enjoyed the book and tried the recipes, please let us know your thoughts.

34904066R00078

Made in the USA
Lexington, KY
29 March 2019